P9-CRD-717

ALREADY TOAST

CAREGIVING AND BURNOUT IN AMERICA

KATE WASHINGTON

Beacon Press
BOSTON

BEACON PRESS
Boston, Massachusetts
www.beacon.org

Beacon Press books
are published under the auspices of
the Unitarian Universalist Association of Congregations.

Printed in the United States of America

24 23 22 21 8 7 6 5 4 3 2 1

This book is printed on acid-free paper that meets the uncoated paper ANSI/NISO specifications for permanence as revised in 1992.

Text design and composition by Kim Arney

Excerpt from "When My Child Fell Ill" by Suzanne Edison from *Michigan Quarterly Review* (Fall 2018). Reprinted with permission.

Library of Congress Cataloging-in-Publication Data

Names: Washington, Kate, author.
Title: Already toast : caregiving and burnout in America / Kate Washington.
Description: Boston : Beacon Press, [2021] | Includes bibliographical references and index.
Identifiers: LCCN 2020030912 (print) | LCCN 2020030913 (ebook) | ISBN 9780807011508 (hardcover) | ISBN 9780807011751 (ebook)
Subjects: LCSH: Caregivers—United States—Psychology. | Women—United States—Psychology. | Burn out (Psychology)—United States.
Classification: LCC HV40.8.U6 W38 2021 (print) | LCC HV40.8.U6 (ebook) | DDC 649.8082/0973—dc23
LC record available at https://lccn.loc.gov/2020030912
LC ebook record available at https://lccn.loc.gov/2020030913

For my daughters, in hopes that our society will be more equitable and caring when they are grown up, and for all the caregivers out there getting through the hard times

CONTENTS

ALREADY
TOAST

INTRODUCTION

COLLATERAL DAMAGE

In despair, I typed "caregiver" into Google, planning to follow it up with "resources" or "support group." The first search the autofill suggested, however, was "caregiver burnout." I sighed and clicked. That morning, I'd cried my way through a miserable appointment with my husband Brad's oncologist. The news we'd received had been no grimmer than any other development over the preceding eighteen months of his treatment for a rare T-cell lymphoma, which had included a debilitating stem cell transplant. But on that hot July day in 2016, I was so exhausted by the caring grind that I could no longer cope. To my embarrassment, I couldn't stop weeping or even look up. I'd always tried to project competence with Brad's physicians so they would take my questions seriously, but by 10 a.m. I was already worn out. I'd spent the morning packing lunches, running our kids to summer camp, loading a heavy wheelchair into the car, wheeling my frail husband across hot asphalt, and picking up a dozen new meds from the Cancer Center pharmacy, all on not enough sleep and with the knowledge that bills, laundry, and plenty else were waiting for me at home. My good-caregiver mask dropped. Tears fell on the coral-colored jersey dress I'd worn to try to present myself as capable rather than a frazzled disaster. As I broke down, the oncologist chided me for not taking good enough care of myself. If I didn't, he said, how could I take care of my husband?

Fragile and overextended, I heard in that question an implication that the only point of me, as a human and not coincidentally as a woman, was to care for another person. What about my own life? Didn't I deserve care in my own right? I left the office as silently as I'd sat in it, but fuming now instead of crying. The so-called self-care that the oncologist had prescribed felt like yet another task I resented, yet another obligation I had to fulfill. What I wanted was for somebody else to volunteer to care for me. Still, I dutifully went home and Googled, intending to look for resources.

The top result for "caregiver burnout" was a quiz to determine whether the caregiver taking it was burned out. I took it. At the end I got the breezy result "You're already toast!" illustrated with a stock photo of a charred piece of bread. The website recommended taking more time for myself, getting a massage or going on walks, arranging for care so I could have an hour to myself, or even an occasional night away. But it said nothing about what to do if I was already doing those things and was burned out anyway.

At first I wasn't particularly bothered by the quiz's cheerful assertion that I was already toast. Toast is the food of invalids, and the food of comfort. The food I turn to when I am sick, when I am sad, when someone I love is either of those things. Cut into strips, soaked in butter, unchallenging, warm, browned, delicious thanks to the Maillard reaction. Why is it also a negative word? Why "you're toast"? Toasting usually makes things better; burning makes them worse. But this quiz result was clearly negative: You're done. Crisped. Eaten. Chewed up. Swallowed. Sounded about right.

I spent more than two years as Brad's primary caregiver during the long, intense crisis phase of his illness; in the years since, as he's endured disability and chronic illness, my responsibilities have ebbed and flowed depending on his health. During the long crisis, I was so overwhelmed, and eventually so burned out, that sometimes I fantasized about simply turning around while driving to the pharmacy or the grocery store, heading to the airport instead, and buying a ticket on any plane going somewhere semitropical. I was forty-two when Brad was diagnosed, and I joked to friends that I was having a very inconvenient midlife crisis, but under the dark humor lay a lot of truth. What stopped me from abandoning my life was the thought of the fallout: Likely endangering my husband's life.

Shocking our friends. Further traumatizing our already fragile children. Inducing lifelong guilt by becoming a person who left her husband at his lowest point. Alienating everyone I've ever loved, everyone who has ever loved me.

I stayed. Brad is no longer desperately ill, but he was permanently disabled by the aftereffects of his treatment. We've worked hard, often painfully, to rebuild our marriage and our lives. It's still a work in progress. In the long ordeal of his illness, his survival was the focus. If cancer is often described as a battle—a metaphor I dislike, since it's hardly a fair fight—I feel like my life was collateral damage.

This book is the story of that toll and of how heavily the weight of caregiving can fall, especially on women. Nobody's caregiving experience will look quite like mine, and this book isn't a traditional how-to resource, but I hope it can prepare people emotionally for the challenges of caregiving or offer solace in the thick of it. Our culture undervalues caring and exploits those who care for others—shunting these tasks disproportionately onto women, people of color, and other marginalized groups, often paying them no more than minimum wage for their efforts. And society often frames family caregiving as both "priceless and worthless," as Evelyn Nakano Glenn puts it in her 2010 book *Forced to Care*.[1] In other words, sentimentalized narratives around caregiving may tell us the work we do is an invaluable gift that is its own reward, as in the very title of the recent book *Priceless Caregiving: Stories of Elder Care Success, Courage, and Strength*. Yet the work of most family caregivers receives little financial support and so lacks economic worth: most family caregivers are never paid, and indeed most take a profound financial hit due to a lack of societal support or of adequate work leave for their role. In truth, however, the work we do has extraordinary economic and social value. Rethinking caring labor in all of its forms, and compensating that labor adequately, is a major issue for contemporary feminism and social justice—one that the coronavirus pandemic laid particularly bare.

This book seeks to bring to light the often hidden phenomenon of caregiving: its invisibility, how American healthcare takes it for granted, how sexism and racism both can drive the assumptions we make about it, how quickly caregivers can burn out, and how urgently we need to change those patterns if we are to build the compassionate, truly caring society that both patients and caregivers deserve.

THE CONSTELLATION OF CARE

Tending to others is at the root of being human. As Arthur Kleinman notes in *The Soul of Care*—his lovely, nuanced portrait of tending to his wife—"care is centered in relationships."[2] So what's the problem with caregiving? In cases of serious illness or ongoing disability, the work of a family caregiver can expand with alarming speed to become a full-time job that includes paperwork and fighting insurance battles, administering IV nutrition and changing colostomy bags, sorting medications and checking insulin.

As a caregiver, I sometimes felt like I barely existed as an individual. One day I had to pick up a prescription for myself and when the pharmacist asked my date of birth, I unthinkingly gave my husband's. I had become so used to providing his birth date that when it was time to meet my own medical needs, I forgot the most basic fact about myself. It was a momentary slip but also a profound moment of erasure. The medication I was picking up was an antidepressant I'd started taking to cope with the anxiety and hopelessness I felt because of someone else's illness. The writer Anne Boyer, in her lyrical memoir of her breast cancer ordeal, *The Undying*, notes how we are intertwined through illness and calls caregiving a kind of suffering in itself: "No patient is sovereign, and every sufferer, both those marked by cancer treatment and those marked by the exhausting routine of caring for those with cancer, is also marked by our historical particulars, constellated in a set of social and economic relations."[3] The constellation of care, illness, and our contingent lives brings us all into webs of care. A disservice to caregivers is equally a disservice to those receiving care.

Caregivers are a huge group. Although hard numbers are difficult to pin down, due to variations in definitions of caregiving, the Family Caregiver Alliance and the American Association of Retired Persons (AARP) estimated in 2020 that 53 million Americans served as unpaid family caregivers, up from 43.5 million in 2015.[4] Additionally, a large "care gap" looms in our future because of the aging of the baby boomers—the oldest members of the generation turn seventy-five in 2021.[5] With birth years 1946–1964, this cohort comprises some 76 million Americans, and its bulk is shifting the overall age composition of the US to skew much older—and more in need of attendance.[6] In our era of sharply declining fertility rates[7] and weaker social ties,[8] that demographic change will leave many people stranded without necessary care.

This coming care gap has pushed caregiving, once all but invisible, into the spotlight as a policy and cultural issue. I was struck recently by a piece in the *New York Times* in which pediatrician Aaron Carroll, who has a regular column, wrote about his experience caring for an ill friend and concluded, "Caregivers aren't supported, and America overlooks their importance."[9] Even for people in the medical field, it's hard to notice the importance of caregivers until you either need one or become one.

AARP has made research and advocacy around caregiving a major focus, ramping up its caregiver support, advocacy, and outreach. I've started to see AARP billboards about caregiving wherever I go, but I first noticed them on a 2018 trip to Palm Springs, where the population is older. An extensive section of the AARP website addressing family caregiving includes legal and medical resources, a caregiver community, tips on life balance, and more.[10] And in a report, the organization calculated the market value of unpaid caregiving work in 2015, aggregating hours worked and calculating the average wage of in-home caregivers or attendants. The resulting figure was a staggering $470 billion.[11] AARP senior strategic policy adviser Lynn Feinberg told me she suspects that even these valuations underestimate the true worth of family caregiving in America, since they include only assistance with daily activities and not skilled nursing tasks, such as administering IV meds.[12] If those tasks were accounted for and the higher wages of nurses applied, the figure would soar even higher.

Because of how the American healthcare system and insurance coverages operate, there's an enormous gap between "too well for the hospital" and "too sick for home." In this gap, in-home care is not covered and the only remaining option is for family members to take over care. In chapter 4, I tell the story of how Brad came home from the hospital after more than four months: visually impaired, immune-suppressed, and so debilitated that his doctors told us he couldn't be left alone even for a minute. His extremely high needs during that time placed a heavy responsibility on me. For the lucky patients, such as my husband, who have good insurance, skilled nursing visits in the home may be covered a few times a week, but that's it. In such situations, family members often sacrifice their work, their personal time, and even their own money to caretaking, a dilemma I examine in more depth in chapter 6.

THE ANGEL IN THE HOUSE

It wasn't just a question of giving care to Brad, though; his illness also meant I took on the entire responsibility of caring for our children, our home, and all the other details of our lives. My mental load as a household manager and my emotional labor as a wife and mother were both heavy during Brad's treatment. In the overwhelming whirlwind of crisis-level illness, I simply did what needed to be done, took help from family and friends despite my tendency toward independence, and paid for what I couldn't manage any other way. An uncomfortable stew of resentment, guilt, and duty simmered beneath the surface every day.

I was among the most privileged of caregivers: I was well off and financially stable thanks to an inheritance from my mother, so Brad's health crisis was not also a financial crisis for us. Brad's job as a unionized university professor, employed by the state of California, meant we had good health insurance, as well as generous leave and other benefits. I was and am a freelance writer, so my work was flexible. We also lived very close to Brad's treatment center and had family help from his parents. Friends stepped up to help keep our daughters on an even keel. My education, social privilege, and even facility in English allowed me to navigate the baffling bureaucracy, understand medical terms and research Brad's condition, wrestle with paperwork, and advocate with doctors. I could even carve out time and money for those massages the caregiving quiz recommended, and I knew I was lucky that all of this was the case.

Yet, even though I had just about all possible advantages and privileges going in, full-time caregiving was all-consuming. It led to extreme stress and burnout, affecting my mental and physical health, relationships, and quality of life. For less privileged caregivers—those with such stressors as financial strain, barriers to good care, and lack of social supports—the challenges become exponential and often crushing. That's bad for caregivers and patients alike—and is an issue of social justice and equity. I wrote this book not just to tell my story but also to advocate for the millions of worried, time-crunched, financially squeezed people caring for others across the United States.

Those pressures are most acute for women, who make up some 75 percent of family caregivers.[13] My experience brought me to a deeper understanding of how unthinkingly our patriarchal culture demands women sacrifice themselves in almost any caring role—and how little it cares about what that does to us. Anne Boyer neatly snapshots the deep, often unconscious layers of care associated with women: "In the waiting rooms, the labor of care meets the labor of data. Wives fill out their husbands' forms. Mothers fill out their children's. Sick women fill out their own."[14] Arthur Kleinman, who focuses on his own growth as a caregiver in his memoir, bluntly points out: "Often, in our society, boys are raised to be careless, girls to be careful." But, he goes on, "while the social pressure and cultural expectations of women to be carers is much greater, it doesn't mean care is natural or easier for them."[15]

The cultural role of caregiving is in many ways an extension of the everyday forms of gender imbalance that exist in heterosexual relationships. Authors and twin sisters Emily Nagoski and Amelia Nagoski, in their book *Burnout*, borrow the concept of "human giver syndrome" from philosopher Kate Manne's book *Down Girl: The Logic of Misogyny* to describe this phenomenon. Manne posits a dual class system, one in which "human beings" have a "moral obligation to be or express their humanity, while human givers have a moral obligation to give their humanity to the human beings"—that is, to "'offer their time, attention, affection, and bodies willingly, placidly, to the other class of people.'"[16] Manne writes: "A giver is then obligated to offer love, sex, attention, affection, and admiration, as well as other forms of emotional, social, reproductive, and caregiving labor, in accordance with social norms that govern and structure the relevant roles and relations."[17] As the Nagoskis put it, "Givers are expected to abdicate any resource or power they may happen to acquire—their jobs, their love, their bodies. . . . Human givers must, at all times, be pretty, happy, calm, generous, and attentive to the needs of others, which means they must never be ugly, angry, upset, ambitious, or attentive to their own needs. . . . If we had set out to design a system to induce burnout in half the population, we could not have constructed anything more efficient."[18] This gender breakdown into "beings" and "givers" is, as Manne herself acknowledges, "far from exhaustive"[19]—and one that leaves out the vast diversity of human experience and relationships. Certainly not all women are subjugated in this manner, and far from all men expect to so subjugate us. This model, however, does offer some illumination of a cultural preconception that operates, I think, unconsciously for many people—and a dynamic I personally experienced: the expectation that caregivers give freely of their entire selves, and more so when we are women.

Once I started noticing caregiving in my own life, it popped up everywhere. Heartbreaking caregiving narratives were there in the novels I'd long loved, such as *Jane Eyre*. Brad and I had met when we were both in graduate school, studying English literature. I worked on Victorian novels; he, on modernism. In the many thick novels I read, I never noticed how many characters were caregivers, dispensing broth to Victorian invalids. But they were there, as they were bound to be in an era when most people died at home. As I entered more deeply into the world of being a so-called cancer spouse, I thought back to them. They were often depicted as little more than shadowy figures in the corner of a darkened sickroom. In fact, one highly gendered model for representation of caregiving dates to this period and trades on a major gender archetype of the era: the Angel in the House, silently bringing soup on a beautifully arranged tray to a delicate invalid and offering full, self-sacrificing support at all times.[20]

The literary caregivers that interested me, though, were more complex. Some were angry, as I have often been angry. Some were neglectful, as I have been tempted to be neglectful. Some were drudges, chained to their charges; others rejected their charges' demands. Some were almost erased, invisible in the narrative, much as I have often felt erased by the demands of being a caregiver.

The parables of caregiving offered by these Victorian and later narratives remain surprisingly relevant, offering insights into the impossibility of the demands still placed on women. It's no accident all these characters were women, despite the obvious existence of male caregivers—the expectation that women will be good at caregiving, due to natural inclination, runs deep.

THE LANGUAGE OF CARE

Care has many senses, but I was surprised to learn the word itself has its roots not in love but in grief. I'd assumed it came from the Latin *caritas*, the root of familiar words such as charity, but no; and there's also no relation to the Latin *cura*, help. Rather, it comes from the Old English *carian*, to grieve, to feel anxious or solicitous, and from the Old High German *charon*, to call out or lament.

Wailing, lamentation, sorrow: these are the roots of caring. There's caring in the sense of loving someone, caring about them; there's also caring in the sense of tending to, caring for them. Caregiving combines the two, with a healthy dose of yet another meaning—the noun meaning "worries," as in, "my cares were heavy."

Give seems more straightforward than *care*: its primary meaning, to bestow or allot, comes from the West Saxon *giefan*, with a secondary definition of yielding to pressure dating to the sixteenth century, and "surrender" (as in give up) to the 1100s. Giving is an act of willing generosity. But I offered that tenderness less freely over time. I had no meaningful choice in giving care: Brad was deathly ill and somebody had to see him through it.

In this book, I use *caregiving* and *caregiver* to refer specifically to caring for ill or disabled people, usually adults.[21] I talk mostly about the kind of caregiver I am—an unpaid family one, doing the work because of relationship ties to the person needing care. Although paid caregiving, and especially how to pay people fairly for this necessary task, is an important element of any consideration of caregiving, it's not the primary subject of this book.[22]

Caregiving can come in many forms, each with distinct attendant challenges. The Caregiver Action Network's website has a kind of choose-your-own-adventure menu for caregivers seeking support, with four basic types of caregivers.[23] There are crisis caregivers, thrust suddenly into the role by acute illness or emergency, as I was when Brad's seemingly indolent form of lymphoma turned suddenly aggressive, a story I tell in chapter 1. Also falling into this category are the four months in 2016 for which he was hospitalized after his stem cell transplant, an acute crisis in which he suffered extreme complications that I describe in chapters 2 and 3. Over the years since then, I've also served as a long-term caregiver—the second type, and a population that's especially vulnerable to burnout, a phenomenon I look at in depth in chapter 5.[24] The third type, long-distance caregivers, live far from their ill or incapacitated charges and must manage their care remotely, a terribly challenging role. Caregiving from afar can often lead to guilt, or may provoke caregivers to worry about whether the care is adequate or they really "count" as caregivers. The fourth category, sandwiched caregivers—which may overlap with any of the others—are those who have other full-time obligations such as a demanding job or young children, and thus are especially pressed for time. I can vouch for how rough the sandwiched life is: our girls were five and nine when Brad was diagnosed. Kids' lives don't stop when a parent gets sick, and though I canceled a lot of piano lessons and allowed a lot of friends to host the girls for sleepovers, I felt overstretched just getting them to school, not to mention soothing their fears about their dad. (For more on what it feels like to be the jam in a caregiving sandwich, see chapter 7.)

There may be clear terminology for all of these kinds of caregivers, but there's no one term that refers easily to all the people they care for—a conundrum that has puzzled me. What's the best way to put it? "The patient," "the sick person," "the object of care," "the loved one" (which sounds like someone has died): none of these quite work. The care-ees are people we caregivers love, and thus neither they nor we are well served by such distancing words as "objects." The relationship between caregiver and cared-for is an emotional, human one and must remain so, if only to stave off the resentment that overstressed caregivers can fall into.

To my mind, the lack of a catchall term underscores the unequal balance between the caregiver and their charge: The recipient of care has a distinct story, subjectivity, a name. The caregiver, by contrast, is almost anonymous—easily hidden by a faceless term. I've seen this in my own life: my husband is the one whose dramatic course of treatment everyone asks about. When he was at his sickest, people asked me, "How's Brad doing?" in the conversational slot where normally they'd have asked, "How are you?" I was support staff who made our family's life run. Brad lost so much in a way so plainly visible to the world; my own losses took place in the background. My daily concerns of, say, washing four laundry loads of sheets drenched by lymphoma night sweats were hardly the stuff of gripping storytelling.

On a more practical level, part of the problem in defining the terminology around those for whom we provide care is their diversity. Some are patients in acute crisis, so "the sick" is an apt term; some are members of the disabled community; some are chronically ill. And the variety of their needs, from assistance with paperwork to injecting medications, compounds the difficulty. I haven't found the perfect way to refer to what the literature often calls *care recipients*, a rather clunky term, so in this book I use "recipient of care," "object of care," or simply "the ill person" interchangeably.

WE ALL NEED CARE

Caregiving strain negatively affects both patients and overstretched families. Its economic and other emotional effects can reverberate for years or decades. As I discuss in chapter 8, putting the pieces back together after caregiving is a challenge that's often overlooked, as caregivers—no less than those for whom they care—can suffer from a form of post-traumatic stress. Everyone should be concerned about how the coming shortfall in caring will affect them, their parents or grandparents, or their children.

Nearly everyone has seen the fallout of the crisis in caregiving: the plight of an elderly neighbor or relative who lives far from children or grandchildren, the friend who must declare bankruptcy after catastrophic medical treatment, even waiting lists for expensive daycare slots for kids all illustrate how thoroughly our society has ignored those who need care. In some ways, the crisis in caregiving for the ill or disabled is an unintended consequence of the success of medical treatment, which has extended the lives of people who in generations past might have died. Brad barely survived a relatively new treatment for aggressive lymphoma; fifty years ago the disease might have killed him before it was ever diagnosed. He deserves better support than what I, his harried wife, could provide alone, and like all caregivers I deserve a life of my own.

For me, care work hardly felt like a vocation, with implications of spiritual purpose and a deep internal longing. Instead, it evoked feelings of obligation. I suspect that's a feeling that many women can identify with, whether because they've been married, a daughter to demanding parents, or a mother. I also worried that I was revealing a deep selfishness because I wasn't intrinsically drawn to the work. Caregiving led me to a much clearer understanding of gender politics and invisible labor not just in my marriage but in my own mind. My new role led to a stark realization of just how much invisible labor—a hot topic in the gender debates in recent years—I had taken on over the course of our marriage. To my surprise, my workload around the house, particularly in matters that touched on organization and the needs of our daughters, did not come close to doubling when I lost my husband's contributions. As Brad's health improved, we faced the daunting task of shifting the balance back. I had to try to explain to him the mental load I'm always carrying. It's required a lot of deliberate communication and commitment to reset our old patterns—sometimes successfully, sometimes not, as I examine in chapter 9.

Arguments about caregiving bump up continually against an impasse. Sick, chronically ill, and disabled people have a right to the care they need to live. Their lives have unquestionable value. The lives and work of we who care for them have value too. But the urgent needs of our charges win out over our own wishes, which can always be deferred to another day, another time. The result is an invisible army of us pressed unwittingly into a kind of service many of us couldn't fully imagine before it crashed into our lives like a sour incarnation of the Kool-Aid Man. I had watched and even helped my mom coordinate end-of-life care for my grandfather, who had Parkinson's disease and resisted the help he needed; even so, I couldn't grasp the all-consuming nature of caregiving until I was in it myself.

For caregivers, the crisis doesn't stop when the immediate threat to life for the ill person ends. In this book's conclusion, I offer a look at ways we could mitigate that damage, but we are a long way from being a truly caring society. The acute emergency of severe, life-threatening illness such as cancer—powerful, expansive, devastating, all-consuming, adrenaline-fueled—is the hurricane. Caregiving is cleaning up after the news crews have left, scrubbing the hidden black mold years later, becoming ill from the contaminated floodwaters. Over the years of Brad's illness, I squeezed in all of the recommended self-care I could—exercise, therapy, occasional time away—but it wasn't enough to meet the ongoing emotional, physical, and logistical demands of the situation. By a couple of years in, I was collateral damage. I was already toast.

ONE

THE LEARNING CURVE

Beginning Caregiving

"Brad is so skinny!" blurted a friend. We were at a wedding and Brad's dress shirt was, indeed, billowing around him, his belt cinched a few extra notches. "Does he have cancer?"

"Of course not," I said, laughing. "He's been going to the gym a lot." But he was in his forties, a time most metabolisms slow, and I too had wondered how he had lost so much weight so fast. I did the cooking in our house, and I knew what he ate. I also went to the gym a lot and I wasn't losing an ounce. Envious, I chalked it up to the unfairly speedy male metabolism.

It was the summer of 2014. He'd lost thirty pounds over the preceding six months, and he's not a big or tall guy. He looked good, taut and wiry. Friends and family exclaimed over how great he looked. But it was just the slightest bit unsettling. A nagging voice in the back of my head had asked, all summer, if he might be having an affair or contemplating one. But I hadn't thought that he might be sick.

My husband's illness sneaked up on us, as did my caregiving role. Our growing understanding of both proceeded as slowly as a watched toaster before startling us like a popped piece of bread. That September, as summer ended, our kids went back to school: Nora, our older daughter, to fourth grade, and Lucy to kindergarten at long last. On their first day, I was relishing the quiet and working at my little desk in our kitchen when Brad came in and offhandedly mentioned some odd lumps along his jawline.

"Do you think I should go to the doctor?" he said, rubbing the beard that had covered his chin for all of the eighteen years I'd known him.

I eyed him. I furrowed my brow.

In the normal we knew before 2014, Brad was a bit of a hypochondriac. His knee would twinge, he would be sure something was sprained or broken, and I'd roll my eyes a little. This time I didn't. I felt his jaw. Indeed, there were weird lumps clustered under his closely trimmed beard. They weren't where a swollen lymph node would be if he were sick. My friend's cancer question floated ominously in my mind. Brad explained that the lumps had been growing.

"At first it was just one and I thought it might be a scar I never noticed before, from when I took that hockey stick in the face," he said. "But now there are more."

I furrowed harder.

"Yes," I said. "I do think you should go to the doctor."

So he did. It took a couple of weeks to get in to see his primary care doctor, as usual. She took some blood tests. His white blood cell counts were a little low, and the lumps were a little odd, but probably nothing, the doctor said. Probably medically unremarkable, as she phrased it: fatty tissue deposits called lipomas, or cysts, or something else. We'd be surprised if it were anything, she said. But if you want, I'll refer you to an oncologist. To be sure.

Brad now says he felt great at the time. In retrospect, I realize he was falling asleep a lot, at odd moments; his energy maybe wasn't as great as he thought. He also got an unusual flu that fall, one in which he had fevers only while sleeping and woke up two or three times a night, the sheets soaked with sweat. Later, we'd learn that night sweats are a telltale sign of lymphoma—a catchall name for a group of blood cancers that affect the immune cells. But he said he was in the best shape of his life. He was playing soccer on weekends, biking to campus to teach his classes as an English professor at Sacramento State, coaching Lucy's soccer team. I was busy with freelance writing work, the girls, and taking care of the million things that need doing in a house and family. Neither of us was thinking we might be facing a medical crisis. For the specialist appointments, Brad shaved his beard for the first time in almost two decades. I posted a picture of him on Facebook with the joking caption, "Married to a stranger!" I didn't know how right I would become.

As he began to see the oncologist, he pushed for answers, with me urging him on from home. It didn't seem like I needed to go to the appointments then. It took a couple of months, but finally someone in oncology agreed to do a needle biopsy of one of the lumps, and we settled in to wait. The fall wore on. I remember talking to a physician friend about the oddness of the waiting, and her reassuring me that it was likely nothing—and that even if it did turn out to be lymphoma, many types never even require treatment. As the holidays inevitably approached, the girls wanted to have a Christmas party, a fancy-dress one. We planned it for the Friday night that school let out for winter break, six days before Christmas, and invited just about everyone we knew. Nora called it our holiday ball, and she made a playlist for it, heavy on the Taylor Swift. I spotted flower-girl dresses in the window of a going-out-of-business bridal shop and bought them, $20 each, for the girls. I made a huge batch of eggnog and used my grandmother's silver punchbowl set for the first time. Our friends came, and we danced and drank until late. Thinking back to that party feels like a distant era, fuzzy and glamorous: the last time we were carefree.

THE WAY WE WERE

The idea of becoming a caregiver was far from my mind as 2014 wound down, even as I pushed away worries about those odd lumps. The main context in which I thought of caring for others was mothering our two girls. Brad, forty-four, had recently wrapped up three years serving as chair of his department at Sacramento State, a job that had made him miserable and done our marriage no favors. He'd started as chair the day Lucy turned a year old, which was also six months after my mother's death by suicide.

When Brad and I had moved to Sacramento for his job, I had resigned myself to caring for my mom in her declining years. She had moved to Sacramento from my smaller hometown, not far away, after I graduated from high school. I never intended to end up back in the Sacramento Valley, but that's where my husband found a tenure-track position. When we relocated, I had to quit my job as associate food editor at a Bay Area–based magazine, and I worried I wouldn't be able to find writing work in the smaller Sacramento area. It turned out, though, that my freelance career thrived. Until the birth of our second child and the death of my mom a few months later, Brad's salary as a professor and my income from freelance writing were roughly on par. I've liked living and working in Sacramento much more than I ever thought I would, but while my mom was still alive, living near her was a mixed blessing. She suffered from bipolar disorder and many other health problems, and our relationship was often fraught. Despite those difficulties, though, the shock of her death, which came shortly before her sixty-fifth birthday, had been devastating. It had driven a wedge between me and Brad: he felt guilty, I felt abandoned when he took a more demanding job in his department shortly after her death, and our sweet baby was among the worst sleepers I've ever encountered, so we were both exhausted all the time. Though I had bitterly grieved and still missed my mom, there was no denying that in some ways her absence was easier than maintaining a relationship with her: no more guilt trips, no more going with her to medical appointments, no more arguing to try to get her to see a new psychiatrist.

By 2014, Brad's and my joint life had settled back down, to the extent that it could, from the upheaval of her death. He was glad to go back to teaching instead of the grind of administration. We were finding our way back to each other. We'd caught up on sleep. We'd made it to the elementary school years for both kids. In the years he'd been chair, I had taken on more and more of the domestic and childrearing labor in our marriage, and gradually our lives had come to look far more traditional: I was handling most household management—including our suddenly changed finances.

My mom's death eased our life in more ways than simply relieving the challenges of a fraught relationship: she left behind an inheritance that boosted our income and enabled me to focus more on the kind of writing I was passionate about, such as creative nonfiction. I still maintained several freelance clients and connections, writing regularly for local and regional magazines, but was now able to turn down work that I had formerly taken for strictly financial reasons. As my writing income dropped, I spent more time managing my mother's estate (a joint project with my brother) and running our household. Though I was still writing, I had less time than I wanted to devote to my work, with creative energy to burn. When Brad's term as chair ended, I had broached the topic of deliberately redressing the balance of labor in our marriage. I didn't want to be responsible for so much at home anymore, and I needed more time and space to revive my professional life in a fresh direction. Finally, as the 2014–15 school year began, it seemed like I might get some breathing room for the first time in years.

By modern standards, Brad and I met and married young. After I graduated from college, I went straight into a doctoral program in my home state of California, which I'd missed terribly while in college on the East Coast. Though he's two years older than I am, Brad arrived at Stanford a year after I did, having taken a fifth year both in high school (then standard in Ontario) and at university, plus a yearlong stop in Toronto to earn a master's degree there. We met at a party, where we bonded over a discussion of obscure 1980s bands. We moved in together ten months later, in part because of the first dot-com boom's pressure on the Silicon Valley housing market.

From the outset, I was more interested in our domestic life: cooking, entertaining, gardening, decorating our minuscule cottage. It had ceilings less than seven feet high, no working heat, and mildewy dampness during rainy California winters. I felt a little bit like the Victorians I studied, working there. We shared the world's smallest office, and I learned quickly to shut my eyes to Brad's teetering stacks of papers and books as I tried to write my dissertation, the idea for which had sprung in part from a casual comment a fellow graduate student had made about *Jane Eyre*. A professor of his, he'd said, had observed that prostitution is "all around the edges" of *Jane Eyre*. The language used to describe Jane, for instance, when she is out on the moors, a woman alone fleeing her bigamous fiancé, is identical to that used to describe sex workers at the time. Jane is a wanderer, alone—like a girl on the streets—and in sexual danger. I was interested, then, in material culture, in the Victorian objects of feminism and women, all of which was the height of academic fashion circa 1995. When I turned to *Jane Eyre*, I got interested in how, after inheriting money, Jane tells her employer (and future husband) Rochester that she is "her own mistress." She also balks, earlier, at Rochester buying her trousseau for their wedding; it makes her feel like a prostitute. I ended up writing about representations of marriage for money versus marriage for love in Victorian literature.

In some convoluted way, all dissertations are autobiographies. Mine, concerning questions of how women might be independent and fulfilled within marriage, was more obviously topical than most, though at the time I missed the connection to my own life. When I wrote it I was in my mid-twenties, living with Brad, wrestling with whether to get married and wondering whether it would be possible to forge an equal marriage. I loved domestic life, wanted to be married, and wanted eventually to have kids. We got married three months before I finished my dissertation. I'd already decided not to seek an academic job. I went into writing and editing instead while Brad forged ahead with his academic career and ended up on the tenure track. Brad never pressured me to leave academia. It was all my choice, born of a mix of factors: I disliked teaching and felt I wasn't good at it (partly because of youthful insecurity); I wasn't sure I had the temperament for academic research; my academic adviser wasn't particularly interested in my work or career; and I wanted to have kids and work part-time. Seeing the stress endured by junior women faculty at my institution made it seem unlikely that I could do those things while staying in the academy. And, underneath it all: I wanted to have those children with Brad. He was a true academic, unwavering in teaching and research as his twin interests, and seemed to be on a fast track, with high-profile advisers invested in him as a candidate. He had no self-doubt that I could see about entering academia, and it seemed unlikely we'd both get jobs if I stuck with it. The job market in humanities was terrible, though it's even worse now.

I've never regretted leaving academia, but I see my choice differently today. I sprinted eagerly into marriage, thinking we had an equal partnership, loving the domestic details of life—but twenty-plus years on, I realize that it was unequal from the get-go, in part because I designated myself as the one who was less professionally driven. I feel now like I walked happily into a trap with my eyes open; in fact, I set it for myself. I grew up in an upper-middle-class, liberal family, my mom a computer programmer. The mainstream-feminist kids' album *Free to Be . . . You and Me* came out the year I was born and played on repeat in my household. Its basic message: as long as you share the housework, you can be whatever you want to be. It seemed that with a little reasonable care to not marry a total asshole and the right kind of communication, I could have a pretty equitable marriage.

I was young, naive, steeped in mainstream white feminism, and I thought equality was there for the plucking. All I had to do was choose the nice guy (check); say I wanted our marriage to be equal (check); choose a career (check); and keep my name (check). I hadn't reckoned with the trap that Ada Calhoun describes so well in *Why We Can't Sleep*, her on-point 2020 book about the particular midlife crisis that my female generational peers and I are having: that being told we could be anything created pressure to *be* everything, without the kind of support that would make it possible. "Women went into the workforce," Calhoun writes, "but without any significant change to gender roles at home, to paid-leave laws, to anything that would make the shift feasible."[1] As she points out, Gen-X women were raised in a bit of a gender-equality paradox: "We're the first women raised from birth hearing the tired cliché 'having it all'—then discovering as adults that it is very hard to have even some of it."[2] Of course, other forces have been at work in the broad inability to have it all: inadequate social supports for needs like childrearing and healthcare, skyrocketing wealth inequality, the shock of the 2008 subprime mortgage crisis, and even, most recently, the coronavirus pandemic all have squeezed the middle class.

My own mom, whose first job out of college in 1967 was with IBM, put her career aside and followed my dad to our small hometown, where she did contract programming work throughout my childhood. I would come home from school to find her at the dining room table with huge green-and-white-striped books of code, but she also did all the housekeeping and nearly all the childrearing. Even though I grew up seeing my mom run the house while my dad went to work, I somehow thought their dynamic was a function of personal choices she'd made a generation before. I overlooked the ongoing structural factors that had conditioned those choices circa 1970—and still did when I got married in 1999. Although my Gen-X friends and I (I should add here that most of my peer group was white and middle or upper-middle class) were hearing and internalizing a rhetoric of equality, I also remember the antifeminist backlash of the 1990s, the struggles over abortion rights (acute at my Catholic university), the Take Back the Night rallies, and the demonization of Hillary Clinton and later Monica Lewinsky. I angrily copied Hillary Clinton's infamous cookie recipe onto a recipe card (which I dug out again to use and share with fellow campaign volunteers in 2016) and wrote furious op-eds for the college paper about campus sexual assault. In the end, though, I retreated from any practical struggle against the broad structures of patriarchal capitalism and into the more theoretical realms of academe—a choice born of privilege and a naive faith that, regardless of broader structures, I could shape my life as I pleased. But by the time Brad had been chair of his department for a year or so, I was shocked at how seamlessly and imperceptibly I'd turned into someone who spent more time as a homemaker than as the writer I had wanted to be. My *Free to Be . . . You and Me*–generation life suddenly looked a lot more like *Leave It to Beaver*. I was determined to shift the patterns back. It still didn't occur to me, then, that I might not be able to make our marriage more equitable by sheer force of will.

LAZY CANCER

A few days after our big, blowout 2014 holiday party came a message sent to Brad's online health portal. It was a result from the biopsy. We both felt anxious, hearts pounding, as he logged in. The result, however, was inconclusive. No cancer cells had been found, but the sample was too small to rule it out. The report, in its dry medical jargon, recommended a core biopsy rather than a fine-needle one. In other words: more limbo, more tests, more uncertainty. We went on with our Christmas—the cracked Dungeness crab and sourdough bread for Christmas Eve, the girls in matching pajamas, presents the next morning—but unease cast a pall over all of it. The girls didn't notice; we had decided not to tell them until we knew something for sure.

Brad went back to the hematologist-oncologist he'd been assigned to, and this time I went with him to ask about the plan. The core biopsy was ordered. We waited, and waited, and waited. Finally, in late February, results came in. Brad indeed had a blood cancer, a type of lymphoma so rare, the doctor said, that it didn't have a name of its own, just a string of markers. We didn't need to know those, the oncologist said. It was too long.

"I've got a pen and a lot of patience," I said. "Try me."

With obvious reluctance, he said: "There's some ambiguity, but we think the best way to describe it is as an indolent non-Hodgkin peripheral T-cell lymphoma, not otherwise specified." Then, a string of cell markers.

"Not otherwise specified" is a catchall term for a group of rare lymphomas; indolent meant it was thought to be slow growing. A word about lymphoma: there are more than seventy types, each with its own distinct treatments and prognosis, and they range from nearly benign (some lymphomas are considered chronic conditions) to aggressively fatal. The two main types are Hodgkin and non-Hodgkin; Brad's was non-Hodgkin (abbreviated as NHL). Most NHLs are B-cells; a smaller proportion are T-cells. Then there are many subtypes of T-cell lymphomas, including the cutaneous (skin) lymphomas Brad's resembled. In general, T-cell lymphomas are not as well understood as other NHLs and are harder to treat, in part because their rarity means there are few clinical trials or opportunities for double-blind studies. I was, of course, Googling madly for all the information I could find about rare lymphomas, treatment options, and what to expect. In this way, the early stages of caregiving played to my strengths: I was good at research, I liked finding out information, I was and am a planner. Learning what we were dealing with, determining next steps, and acting as an advocate, while also supporting Brad emotionally—all of this was scary but didn't seem onerous. With my pen and notepad, pushing the oncologist for more answers, I could feel like I was in control, succeeding at this new job. Much as I'd experienced with marriage itself, I didn't realize how hard it would be later, as the glow wore off and the challenges ramped up.

Brad's oncologist assured us that, because his disease was indolent, it was not particularly urgent to treat it. Some of the most common forms of lymphoma never require treatment or turn dangerous, he said. The plan for now, he said, was watch, wait, and research potential treatment options. He seemed reluctant to treat at all.

We left the office. We joked that Brad had lazy cancer. I still wasn't thinking much about what it might mean to care for him. Of course, I knew that his cancer would affect our lives, but at that point it was still possible to be in denial about how much.

The weekend after the diagnosis was the fifth anniversary of my mother's suicide. My in-laws were in town visiting, and we drove to my hometown for the day. I'm close with my brother, and on the anniversary of our mom's death we try to get together. Late February also happens to be when the almond trees in northern California are in bloom, so we often meet up at my dad's almond farm for a picnic during what's usually a small break of springlike weather.

Brad was tired and coughing a lot on that day trip. We went to my brother's house, where the girls played with their younger cousin. Brad lay down on the couch, wrapped a blanket around himself, and nodded off. I looked over at my mother-in-law and there were tears in her eyes.

"He looks so sick," she said. "It feels like I'm looking into the future." She shivered.

I saw her point. He was pale, crumpled, gaunt: a harbinger of worse times to come.

Brad's oncologist was of the old-fashioned type and seemed unsettled when we pushed back on the "let's not do anything" plan. He finally, reluctantly, offered a plan for chemo with a drug more commonly used as a second-line treatment; our insurance denied the claim on that ground. Brad and I had many agonized conversations about that; I remember discussing potentially paying for it out of pocket, even though nobody was particularly convinced it would be effective. We asked for a second opinion at Stanford, where the medical center has a specialty clinic that treats cutaneous lymphomas. Brad's didn't quite fit, but they were interested in his case. He was, we were already learning, that unlucky patient to whom doctor after doctor would say, "We've really never seen this before."

Stanford wanted to run some additional tests, including a bronchoscopy (running a camera into Brad's lungs) to see why he might be coughing so much. Looking back, it's unclear to me why nobody ever suggested a PET scan, the gold standard for cancer detection. Brad was known to have tumors on his jawline and abdomen, and lymphoma is a systemic cancer. If I'd known then what I know now as a caregiver, I'd have fought tooth and nail for a PET, something I've had to do on occasion since then. But I was still naive and still not fully accustomed to acting as a patient advocate. So we waited. I remember that Brad's coughing increased in severity that spring. With some trepidations about whether we should travel far from our usual medical care, we took the girls to Hawaii on a spring-break trip we'd planned before Brad's diagnosis. A friend who knew about the diagnosis but whom I hadn't seen for a while later told me that when she saw our pictures on Facebook she wondered if it had been the kind of trip you take when everything's about to change. We hadn't planned it that way, but it was absolutely that kind of trip.

IN WHICH EVERYONE IS SURPRISED

A few weeks after we got home from that trip, we were having a normal Saturday. I'd done some gardening, pulling out the last of the winter's kale and overgrown spinach. I found a dead rat under our grapefruit tree. Brad disposed of it, to my relief. For dinner I grilled chicken and served it with those leftover vegetables. I was sitting at the table with the girls, irritated with Brad for delaying dinner—it often took him what seemed like ages to get a drink and get to the table—and equally irritated with the girls, who were pestering me about repainting their nails, which I'd already done and they'd promptly ruined.

He called me from the bathroom. "Hang *on*," I snapped.

"No," he said urgently between coughs. "Come *now*."

This was real, I realized, my adrenaline spiking. Blood was splashing out of his mouth, blooming over the white porcelain of the sink. The splashes coming up out of his throat made little noises, like the gurgle of an unstuck drain. It was a lot of blood, with more coming. Each time he coughed it seemed like a half cup. I grabbed a bucket from the broom closet and handed it to Brad and then ran across the driveway to our neighbor Chet's back door and banged on it. Chet opened the door, alarmed at my urgency.

"Can you come over and stay with the girls? I have to take Brad to the emergency room," I panted. "There's dinner. Eat whatever you want."

He agreed. I don't know why we didn't call an ambulance, except that I thought I could get Brad to the UC Davis Medical Center ER faster myself, and I wanted to go with him. We both thought he might be dying. The streets were deserted, bathed in the golden light of a May evening. I honked my horn and rolled right through the two red lights I hit between home and the ER. Brad continued to disgorge thick blood into the bucket.

At the ER, I quickly learned the word for what was happening: hemoptysis, which is simply fancy medical speak for coughing up blood. It took a few more days to learn what had caused it. In the confusion of his first few days in the huge teaching hospital that our medical center runs, one thing became clear: neither the lung guys nor the cancer guys wanted him as their patient. The pulmonologists told us they suspected the blood had come from a ruptured lung tumor. The oncologists, for their part, thought it was an injury from the bronchoscopy two weeks previously. A CT scan settled the question: a tumor, which had grown rapidly on a blood vessel deep in the lung, had indeed ruptured. Brad's lymphoma was much more aggressive than anyone had suspected, and the bronchoscopy had missed the tumor only because it was at the far corner of his left lung. There was no more talk about indolent cancer; he needed chemo urgently.

This episode plunged me directly, and unexpectedly, into intense caregiving. I was stretched between the hospital and home, trying to advocate for my husband to two different sets of doctors in the complex, opaque bureaucracy of a major teaching hospital. Brad's oncologist, the doctor we knew, practiced only in the Cancer Center, not the main hospital, so he was impossible to reach, and I was angry at what seemed like his callousness and lack of involvement. Rounds by the various doctors—the only chance to get information and ask questions—seemed to have no schedule, except that they invariably occurred five minutes after I absolutely had to leave to go to the bathroom or pick up my daughters from school. Soon, however, Brad was transferred to the oncology floor—where, as it turned out, he would spend a full half of the year that followed.

Early in that hospital stay, I got a first glimpse of the scope of family caregiving. Brad needed chemo urgently, and for that, the doctors told us, he needed a PICC (peripherally inserted central catheter)—an IV line, semipermanently placed in his arm, that would lead to his heart. Communication in the hospital being what it was, we learned of this only when the IV specialist nurse showed up bedside to get informed consent to place the PICC. There was just one issue: Brad had a needle phobia and was so squeamish he couldn't stand any talk of blood, especially if it involved veins or the heart. I'd seen his needle phobia in action before, shortly after Nora was born. Because we'd had a baby, we were applying for life insurance, an optional benefit through his work, and it required a basic physical for each of us. The company's policy was to send a traveling nurse to our home to do the physical, which required a blood draw. I had mine done and stood by holding the baby during Brad's turn. Within seconds of the needle going in his arm, he'd turned pallid and slid under the table. He came to, swearing at us both, as I hastily put Nora into her crib and tried to help the nurse haul him up. (He was a terrible candidate for a blood cancer, really, though over the past few years exposure has greatly lessened the phobia.)

The PICC placement was a far more delicate procedure than a simple blood draw, and I knew that he would decline it if he thought he could. Without it, though, he couldn't get the chemo he needed. I motioned the nurse outside. "So how much information does he need to consent?" I asked. "It would be best if you didn't mention veins, the heart, or the needle at all." She gave me a look, but she soft-pedaled the explanation, and I followed up by saying to Brad that I would read to him through the whole procedure to distract him. I felt a bit like Jem Finch reading aloud to the detoxing Mrs. Dubose in *To Kill a Mockingbird*.[3] As the nurse prepped Brad's arm, I held his other hand and read steadily from a favorite book of his, *The Irish R.M.*[4] He focused on my voice so the needle wouldn't make him faint. The procedure took an hour, and afterward the nurse complimented me for keeping Brad steady and helping her get consent. The moment drove home for me the importance of family caregivers: sometimes, you have to really know a person to understand what kind of care they need. For another patient, fudging the consent and reading an obscure humor book would be exactly the wrong approach; for my husband, it was the only answer.

Brad was transferred to the oncology ward and started chemo the day after the PICC went in. The chemo worked almost too well—the lung tumor shrank so fast it left a hole in his lung, which collapsed and filled with a toxic fluid. Brad's oxygen levels dropped, the pulmonologists weren't sure how to proceed, and there was talk of admitting him to the ICU. By the time he'd been inpatient for a week, I was already worn out from spending long hours at the hospital, communicating with family and friends, taking care of the girls and doing everything that needed doing around the house. At the time, we had a very badly behaved cat, and I remember getting home from the hospital one hot night only to find the cat had escaped and was hiding under our deck. I had to crawl through dead leaves and old spiderwebs to extricate him—the last straw in a long day. I was already noticing, however, that Brad's absence hadn't added much to the things I needed to do around the house. In fact, it subtracted a certain amount of tidying up, reclosing of cabinet doors, and similar tasks, since I like a neat house and Brad could not care less.

Caregiving often pushed me into more traditional feminine roles, especially in outward forms of self-presentation. I tried to show up at the hospital in a nice outfit, often a dress, and lipstick so I would look put-together and competent. I tried to seem intelligent, hoping for a measure of respect. I was often disappointed.

Often I felt like the doctors didn't even see me as an independent person. On one particularly stressful day, it seemed like Brad might need to be transferred to the ICU because his lung had collapsed and his oxygen saturation was low. Scared, I asked a resident about these concerns and when we might see the pulmonologists. She stonewalled me hard, talking down to me in response to every question, frequently interjecting what she assumed was my name—presumably as a way to help soothe me and make me feel seen. But she'd never asked my name. Instead, she was calling me "Mrs. Buchanan"—Brad's last name, which I've never used. She brushed me off, over and over, with variations on, "What you have to understand, Mrs. Buchanan, is . . ."

Finally, I stopped her. "My name isn't Buchanan," I said. "And you're condescending to me. I'd appreciate it if you would at least call me by my name when you do it."

She was flustered, but I was too mad to feel bad about it. "What . . . what would you like to be called?" she asked.

"You may call me Kate," I said, "or you may call me Dr. Washington." I've never used my doctorate as a title, either socially or professionally. I'd earned it, but, as I haven't pursued an academic career, using it usually feels pretentious. (I use Ms. instead.) In this case, though, I felt like being obnoxious. I regretted it afterward, especially when Brad told me I shouldn't have fought with a resident. But I don't regret correcting her assumption about my name. A friend of mine in medicine later told me that medical students are still always trained to call family and patients by an honorific and last name, but in this case that training led to an assumption that was sexist, even though it was made by a woman. It would have been easy to ask what I wanted to be called. That resident, of course, never called me anything again and avoided me as much as possible, as I did her.

Another hidden aspect of my role in the family and as a caregiver was what sociologists call "kin work": in this case, keeping family and friends up to date on the crisis. More broadly, this kind of labor, often performed by women, includes building family and social ties through things such as birthday and Christmas cards, gifts, or traveling to see relatives. Such work may not seem like an obvious part of care, and for many of us it's so ingrained that it's hard to see it as labor, but it's a necessity that adds to the caregiver's load—and, as I quickly found, it can be more than a little fraught. Especially in the case of informing Brad's parents, far away in Canada, I felt caught between my husband, who wanted to downplay the severity of his illness so as not to worry them, and their right to know what was happening. Brad and I argued about this, especially because his mother wanted to come help and at first he didn't want her to.

At the end of that first week in the hospital, however, he was sick enough that he cracked and asked me to ask her to come. I sent an email late that night, California time, to her in Ottawa. By the time I woke up at 6 a.m. Pacific—it happened to be Mother's Day—she was getting on a plane. The relief I felt at her arrival, late that day, was enormous.

When Susan arrived it felt like I had an ally for the two remaining weeks Brad stayed on Davis 8, the hospital floor to which he would eventually return and spend months. She was a reassuring presence and when Brad came home she became a sounding board for how to manage with a fragile patient in the house. What I later came to think of as the cloven pine of caregiving hadn't yet closed around me. In the early days of intense emergency I still felt like myself, and Brad still seemed like himself. The crisis seemed temporary. As the balance of our relationship shifted, I would come to feel more and more isolated, but at the time, I foolishly thought Brad was about as sick as he would get. The emergency had been frightening but now, I believed, would come the stable phase of treatment, to be followed by remission. I never realized how much sicker he could get yet still survive.

SUMMER OF CHEMO

While Brad was in the hospital we became disillusioned with his oncologist, who had been uncommunicative throughout his hospitalization and who still hadn't outlined a clear treatment plan. I was talking with some acquaintances at my gym, where word had gotten out that my family was in the midst of a crisis. (Later, my workout buddies would rally to bring us meals for weeks on end.) One woman happened to be a pharma rep, selling one of the rare chemo drugs that the doctors were considering for Brad. We got to talking about our discomfort with the oncologist and the sense that he wasn't really up to date on Brad's case. She offered the cell number of another oncologist in the same group, one who specialized in rare lymphomas such as Brad's.

I felt strongly that Brad needed better care and a clearer plan of action. It was already evident that his cancer wasn't following a predictable narrative. But as he was still weak and still in the hospital, I didn't want to take advantage of his condition to push a change he didn't want himself. For me it was an early test in the ethics of caregiving, where sometimes the judgments of the patient and the caregiver may not entirely align. In that case, who wins? Wary of overstepping, I talked to Brad about the credentials and background of the potential new doctor. To my relief Brad was enthusiastic, and Dr. T, as I'll call him, was immediately responsive and interested in Brad's case, visiting him in the hospital. Brad is now sure Dr. T saved his life more than once, and credits me with that.

Before Dr. T could begin more treatment, though, Brad first had to recover at home from his initial dose of chemo—the huge blast that had filled his lung with toxic fluid. Although he was well enough to come home after nineteen days, the doctors judged that he wasn't well enough to get more chemo on the usual three-week cycle. And when they resumed the chemo treatments they were all done inpatient, via a long, slow drip that lasted for four days—a safety measure to prevent another extreme reaction like the collapsed lung.

As eager as we both were for Brad to get treated, the reasons for the delay were easy to understand. He came home in late May badly weakened and visibly ill, with high treatment needs at home. He'd lost more weight and color in the hospital and he moved slowly. He also came home on oxygen and ultra-strong IV antibiotics—his lung was still filled with a thick fluid and was at high risk of serious infection. I was floored when I learned that I was expected to administer these antibiotics three times a day, through his PICC line. In addition to that he came home with a complex regimen of well over a dozen medications, and it fell to me to fill his extra-large pill box and refill his prescriptions.

At the time of discharge, he was eager to get out of the hospital, but I was concerned they were sending him home too soon and was uncomfortable with how discharge decisions got made. Discharge is its own vast world in the opaque, complex bureaucracy of the hospital, which comes as a surprise to many patients and families—as it did to me. What I found was that discharge personnel were often only tenuously connected with the medical staff I'd dealt with while Brad was inpatient. In many cases, the new discharge coordinators and their minions were actually outside consultants, not hospital staff, and they were generally unfamiliar with Brad's case. The providers training me were not the nurses and doctors we'd come to trust but traveling practitioners from an external contracting company with whom I had no rapport—and who obviously needed to fill daily quotas to train as many caregivers as they could.

That nurse in this case spent about half an hour training me how to keep my husband alive and left me nervous and unsure about my ability to do so. My concern was a common one. In recent decades the medical establishment has increasingly outsourced relatively complex at-home care tasks to family caregivers, often with little training. When skilled nursing tasks become the province of the caregiver, training is often minimal. A report issued by AARP, "Home Alone," sharply criticizes this widespread practice: "A health care system that relies on untrained and unpaid family members to perform skilled medical/nursing tasks, but does not train and support them, has lost sight of its primary mission of providing humane and compassionate care to sick people and their families."[5] The report urges healthcare providers to "fundamentally rethink and restructure the way they interact with family caregivers in daily practice."[6]

Just as I didn't realize what would be expected of me until Brad was sent home, few know what's coming with higher-level caregiving. The early days of caregiving often felt to me like the newborn period with my first baby: I'd been sent home from the hospital with something fragile and precious and I couldn't believe they thought I could manage its needs. As with a baby, there's a steep learning curve to caring for a fragile patient, and often family caregivers get most or all of their understanding from trial and error, as a recent piece in *Forbes* points out: "Family caregivers often provide assistance with love and compassion, but no skills. That lack of training makes their lives more difficult and makes it more likely that those they are caring for will fall, get infections, or suffer from dehydration or malnutrition."[7] A bumbling or incompetent caregiver—or even a well-intentioned but inexperienced one like me—can be dangerous for patients, and the stress on the caregiver in such a situation is also considerable. I'm not alone in feeling underqualified for such tasks: one study showed that 93 percent of family members caring for an elder said they've never been taught how to be a caregiver.[8]

SALINE FLUSH

For three weeks after Brad came home our days were marked by the ritual of administering his IV antibiotics at regular eight-hour intervals: 6 a.m., 2 p.m., 10 p.m. Here were the steps: first, I washed my hands with hot water and antibacterial soap (crucial for an immune-compromised chemo patient), fingertips to midforearm, rinsed, and turned off the tap with a dry elbow. I walked with hands held high. I avoided thinking about how I never used to buy antibacterial soap because it creates drug-resistant super bacteria.

Second, I unwrapped the saline, the antibiotic, the second saline, the heparin, and the orange line cap and laid them on a plastic tray. I dealt out alcohol wipes like tiny cards in a grim game of solitaire. I had to let go, quickly, of any qualms about waste and the environment in my new life as an overwhelmed caregiver. The nurse who trained me said that when she gave her spiel about how to administer IV antibiotics in a neighboring ultraliberal college town, she had to start by telling people they couldn't think about the environment right now. I emptied the wastebasket by Brad's bed daily; it filled up fast with syringes, wrappers, line caps, empty Ensure bottles, tissues, and paper plates from toast I brought downstairs to the guest room where Brad was set up during his convalescence. I slept alone in our king bed upstairs, sticking neatly to my side even though nobody else was there, and used the often-messy bathroom shared with our daughters while Brad had a clean guest bath to himself. In the guest room, an oxygen tank bubbled nearby and an enormous stack of sheets lay ready for the night sweats his cancer caused. The piles of sweaty sheets every morning and the full wastebasket were the detritus of cancer, an outward metaphor for the chemotherapy's unseen work inside his body, the cleaning and expelling of waste cells.

Third, I twisted the white cap off the first saline syringe, pulled the plunger down, and pushed it up to expel the air. I held it upright and pulled the plunger down, just a millimeter, pushing up to expel the air. A drop of saline beaded—like a tear, its meniscus bulging—on the surface.

Most days I blinked, hard, as another kind of saline swelled at the corner of my eye.

"Don't worry," Brad said on the first night, when I was trying not to shake, terrified of leaving air in the line and trying desperately to remember everything the nurse had said. "The nurses in the hospital sent the saline flying," he said with a smile. I thought suddenly of the title of a George Orwell novel, *Keep the Aspidistra Flying*, and in an instant our shared past swam up. I tried not to think about how we met, how different he had become, our likely future. I tried not to send the saline flying from the meniscus in my eye. The times when it spilled over, I couldn't wipe my eyes; I had to keep my hands sterile. The tears trickled down the side of my nose, irritatingly. (After a few days I gained confidence and occasionally sent the saline flying myself, breaking the seal one-handed, squirting a bit up in the air as if this were a medical drama on TV. But I was wearing pajamas, not scrubs, and I was no nurse.)

Next, I tore open a tiny alcohol-wipe packet and rubbed the wipe hard around the threads for his PICC line. I tried not to worry that I might somehow have missed a spot or touched something or insufficiently cleaned the line or introduced bacteria that could snake up the tiny tubes straight to his heart. I tried not to think about what my brother and father—both attorneys who defend clients in medical malpractice cases—had told me about how bad it can be if those lines get infected. I rubbed the tiny wipe over the line end again and flicked it into the quickly filling trash can. I twisted the saline syringe onto the line and depressed the plunger in delicate little pushes so that saline flowed into the line.

I mustered a smile every time Brad said, "Refreshing!" as the saline flowed into his vein, cool like ocean water. Mostly I did find this small attempt at lightening the moment amusing, endearing. Sometimes, though, I was tired or worried or thinking about the four laundry loads of night-sweat-drenched sheets waiting after the 6 a.m. meds or battling the hot saline in the corner of my eye, and I would rather have skipped the banter. (Brad was having drenching night sweats up to five times a night. I made frantic trips to Ikea and Target for waterproof mattress liners and absorbent jersey sheets, and begged friends who offered to help to pick up fragrance-free detergent. Susan and I finally realized we should make the guest bed lasagna-style, alternating fitted sheets and waterproof liners so Brad could strip away layers through the night. This produced about four loads of laundry every day—and it takes jersey sheets forever to dry. That's when I started sending out the laundry twice a week—but the sight of that mountain of laundry every morning still gave me a moment of fresh dread.)

After the saline, after another alcohol wipe, I attached the crucial antibiotics and pushed them, one milliliter every twenty seconds, slowly: five to ten minutes for the syringe. Each milliliter was a tiny, resistant depression with the thumb, the antibiotic more viscous than the saline. I resisted the temptation to push harder so I could drink my coffee before the kids woke up or get on with my day or get to bed sooner.

After the antibiotics I repeated the alcohol wipe, the saline, the alcohol wipe. I pushed in blue-capped heparin to keep the line from clotting and clamped the line. I twisted on the little orange SwabCap, which includes an alcohol-soaked pad to keep the line sterile and fit tight on the plastic threads. Feeling its snug twist was the most satisfying moment of the whole procedure.

Three times a day I gently nested the flexible plastic line ends on Brad's too-thin, too-pale arm and pulled on a mesh sleeve to protect the tubing and his fragile vein. "All done," I said, turning off the light so he could return to sleep. Three times a day I returned the striped plastic tray, empty, to the bar where we used to host parties. Three times a day I thought about how quickly, how completely, everything in our life had changed, and I again felt the saline meniscus in my eye.

Six, two, ten. Three times a day. The stress of providing complex care for which I had been only briefly trained was extreme. At the same time, performing those nursing tasks—once I got over the fear I would kill my husband—was what made me feel like a "real" caregiver.

There was a subtle officious pleasure, then, in the ritual of administering the antibiotics. I knew exactly why I was doing it; I understood precisely how I was contributing to my husband's continuing life, preventing infection with a specialized task I had learned. The crisis was fresh, my energies and compassion still undrained, the grinding weight of caregiving not yet so heavy and ambiguous as it became later. We thought then that he would recover from this crisis, undergo routine chemotherapy, go into remission, and recover. Then, I still basked in a false sense of certainties and clarities around caregiving: if I do this well, if I inject the antibiotics at the right times, if I keep everything sanitary, if I understand the doctors, if I earn an invisible gold star, I will contribute to his recovery, and life can settle back into its expected shape.

IN WHICH EVERYONE IS SURPRISED AGAIN

It didn't happen that way. Brad went through his summer of treatment: he went to the hospital every three weeks for five days of boring inpatient chemotherapy. I traveled with the girls to our family cabin in a remote part of the Sierra Nevadas above my hometown, ran them to camps and play dates, and threw their summer birthday parties. Nora, turning ten in July, begged for a slumber party; I held it in a hotel because Brad was coming home from chemo on her birthday and the thought of cleaning up after five girls before he got back sounded impossible. Lucy wanted a national park–themed party, bafflingly, for her August birthday. Her original idea was that I dress up in a ranger outfit and set up an installation on the front lawn (we didn't have a backyard then). I couldn't quite wrap my mind around that, so instead I booked picnic tables at a nature center on the American River, where real rangers could do an ecology presentation, complete with owls. Brad was able to come, and I remember his striking pallor.

Throughout that summer, once Brad's course of antibiotics was over, he didn't need much direct care from me, but I was caring for everything else, especially during his long, dull stretches of hospitalization. The girls and I traveled to pass the time while he was inpatient; it was often easier and more fun to manage them away from home. When Brad wasn't in the hospital he was taking long walks, often through a nearby cemetery.

He finished chemo over Labor Day weekend. To our relief his doctor pronounced him in remission. The next step in Dr. T's plan was to prep him for an autologous stem cell transplant—a relatively low-risk procedure using his own bone-marrow stem cells, harvested in advance, to replace his bone marrow, the organ that was producing the cancerous T-cells. It would be unpleasant, but using his own stem cells meant there was no risk of the rejection called graft-versus-host disease, which can happen with donor stem cells in the other type of transplant, called allogeneic. In both types of transplant, chemo and radiation are used in ultrahigh doses to wipe out the existing marrow and take the patient down to zero immunity; the patient must then receive a graft of new stem cells to repopulate the marrow, or they will die.

The evidence was relatively weak that autologous transplants could cure cancers of Brad's type. It seemed a lot better, though, than doing nothing and waiting for a relapse, which Dr. T seemed pretty sure would come without additional treatment. And with Brad's cancer, the evidence for everything was weak, as I learned when I Googled lots and lots of medical journal articles about T-cell cancers, trying to learn more. During that period—after chemo, before the transplant—I didn't think of myself much as a caregiver. I Googled a lot, provided emotional support, ran the household, but I was no longer administering IV medications or filling the pillbox.

Our questions around the autologous transplant turned out to be irrelevant; Brad never underwent the procedure. A few weeks after finishing chemo he said he could feel those lumps again on his abdomen and jaw. Dr. T was skeptical, saying it would be extremely surprising if the cancer had relapsed so fast. But we pushed for a PET scan, which confirmed a very aggressive return of the cancer. The results came on my forty-third birthday, so we spent a very glum dinner date discussing the news and his options, which were few. Really the only hope of survival, Dr. T said, was a far riskier allogeneic stem cell transplant, which uses stem cells from a donor. A suitable donor would need to be found as soon as possible. In the meantime Brad went on a second-line chemo to try to knock back the disease as much as possible before transplant—and I started learning more about what we were up against.

TRANSPLANT PREP

That fall of 2015 was a time of keyed-up limbo. The first order of business was to talk to Brad's only sibling, James, about whether he could be a donor. A sibling has a one in four chance of being a match, so it wasn't assured by any means, but transplant teams prefer to use sibling matches whenever possible. James lives in Canada so he had to fly in for testing and vetting. If James proved not to be a match, the transplant service would move on to checking the donor registry. Feeling helpless, I registered, even though there was a vanishingly small chance I'd be a match for Brad. Registering is a simple process—it requires only a simple cheek swab—and for someone who needs a match, a donation, now relatively noninvasive, can be lifesaving.[9]

The quick reversal of Brad's fortunes was hard to explain, and I felt increasingly removed from our friends. During Brad's earlier hospitalization, we got a lot of support from friends who ran a Meal Train and went on errands, but I knew we were likely to need a lot more before all this was over, so I shrank from asking for too much too soon. At the same time, the withdrawals of some people who had previously said we were like family stung; others stepped up unexpectedly and became new friends, but it took a long time.

Socializing was often awkward. I remember a get-together with some women friends, all of whom were terribly sorry for what I was going through. They talked about birthdays, drank wine, shared about their kids. I mostly stayed quiet; it never seemed like the right time to explain how dangerous the transplant would be or the technical challenges of it, but one friend—a physician—started grilling me about the plans, suggesting maybe they weren't the best option. Then the whole group took up the subject of registering as a donor. I was explaining to them what a long shot it is—one chance in millions—for anyone who's not related to turn out to be a match. But, as I've done often since, I encouraged those friends to get on the donor registry. A friend who may have had a couple of glasses of wine said, "Well, can I just register to donate to Brad? I mean, I'd be happy to help him, but I wouldn't want to have to donate to just anybody." I don't think she'd thought about the implications of what she was saying but my first reaction was to wonder what if, somewhere out there, Brad's match was saying the same thing to another patient's caregiver. After that, I avoided groups where I might feel equally out of step.

It's hard to find clear survival rates for those receiving transplants, as the factors involved (which transplant center was used, age at time of transplant, type of underlying disease) can vary so widely, but at the time I was seeing survival rates of about 65 percent—a number that sounds kind of okay until you flip it and realize it means 35 percent of people getting a transplant die. Brad's doctor assured us that Brad, being relatively young and not too debilitated going in, had better odds than most. I had our will and trust documents updated anyway. Brad, who had been walking all over the neighborhood to stay active during his treatment, also wanted to buy crematory niches at a cemetery near us, so we did that too. I think we startled the woman working there; Brad was wearing a hat, so you couldn't tell he was a cancer patient, and they apparently don't get a lot of healthy-looking fortysomethings walking in off the street to buy cemetery real estate. We had some moments of grim humor: when she asked if we wanted to look at in-ground niches, Brad said no on the grounds that he'd seen too many people walking their dogs there and he didn't want to be peed on for eternity.

Some of our stress was eased when we learned that James was a match. The days went by. Christmas came, and that year brought with it no blowout party. In the past we'd gone to Canada to visit Brad's family for the holidays in odd-numbered years. That wasn't possible in 2015 with him still undergoing chemo and susceptible to infection. We stayed home.

Brad surprised us all, even me, with a combination pool and ping-pong table for our basement. He had somehow smuggled it downstairs piece by piece and he spent hours on Christmas Eve assembling it. His idea was that it would be a good indoor activity for his recovery.

Our New Year's Eve was subdued. In fact, I don't remember anything about it—it's always been one of my least favorite holidays. What I do recall is how we spent January 2, 2016, the day before Brad went into the hospital: we took the girls to a matinee of the latest Star Wars movie, *The Force Awakens*, which had just come out, and went out for a last family dinner at our favorite restaurant, a neighborhood pizza joint called One Speed that opened around the same time Lucy was born. Going there the night before Brad went into the hospital for chemo had become a mini tradition over the preceding summer, and it was bittersweet that night. Brad wouldn't go to a restaurant again for many months and he still hasn't been back to a movie theater. I would say it was the last normal-feeling day we would have as a family, but even at the time it didn't feel normal. We were on a knife's edge, all too keenly aware of how everything was about to change.

TWO

THE THICK OF IT

BMTU, Part One

Brad entered the hospital to begin pre-transplant care on January 3, 2016. That morning, a Sunday, was strange and anxious. My dad drove to Sacramento to stay with the girls while I took Brad to the hospital. He was packed and ready. Brad was sure, so sure, that he would be home in thirty days—the minimum hospital stay for a transplant if everything went perfectly. I, doubtful, was worried that he was too optimistic and would be devastated later if things didn't go as well as he expected. I'd experienced his balloon-like optimism before. He would maintain a buoyant attitude as long as he could, but when some setback inevitably popped it, he tended to plunge into the depths of despair. As a caregiver I wanted a middle path of realism that was neither pessimistic nor optimistic, that took all of the possibilities into account, enabling me to plan for contingencies. Our divergent attitudes were a frequent source of tension.

On that Sunday morning I got a quick glimpse of the fragility of his positive outlook. At the hospital, where everything moves at its own slow pace, things were in disarray. The bone marrow transplant unit (BMTU), a separate wing of the familiar oncology ward with private isolation rooms, was full. A patient hadn't yet been discharged so they didn't have a room for Brad. They could put him in a small room on the regular oncology ward and move him when a room in the BMTU proper opened up. Brad's mood turned immediately dark; I moved into soothing his frustration, reassuring him that it would be okay, that he'd get the right room. It wasn't easy to talk him down and it felt like the whole enterprise was getting off to a bad start. He'd heard in advance he could have an exercise bike in his room if he asked but there wasn't space in the cramped substitute room. He wasn't sure if he should unpack the things he'd brought—books and research materials for an academic project he was working on intermittently. Privately I thought he was overly optimistic to bring them and to assume he'd be on an exercise bike daily, but I kept that thought to myself. I was learning that part of caregiving was knowing when and whether to share my opinions.

There really wasn't anything to do at the hospital. Nothing was happening with Brad medically on that first day; it felt strange to bring a man who seemed basically well to the hospital and leave him there. I wasn't sure whether I belonged at home with the kids or at the hospital with Brad. Once I'd talked him down from his rage about the room foul-up we didn't have much to say. During the week ahead he was slated to receive intensive chemo and full-body irradiation. In an allogeneic stem cell transplant, the goal is to first blast the body with as much chemo and radiation as it can take, killing all the existing bone marrow so that the patient can't grow any new white blood cells. Once the white blood cell count is at zero—a terrifying number to see on a chart—the donor's bone marrow stem cells are dripped in steadily through an IV transfusion. The hope is that they will take hold and eventually begin manufacturing new white blood cells, a process called engraftment.

A stem cell transplant, though it sounds clean and coolly technical, is brutal. If the donor backs out or if engraftment doesn't occur, the patient, now with no immunity whatsoever, will die. The preparatory chemo and radiation are administered at far higher doses than normal, a scorched-earth tactic that takes the patient close to death. In the days leading up to the transplant Brad developed painful mouth sores, lost all his hair, and contracted C. diff colitis.[1] Soon, his airy hopes of using the exercise bike and working on his research vanished with his appetite.

While Brad was getting preliminary treatment at the hospital I was getting ready for James to come to town to make his donation, and then for Brad's parents to arrive after that. Joe and Susan planned to stay as long as needed, to help on both the home and hospital fronts. It was invaluable support but came with a certain amount of emotional strain. Looking back at my calendar I see that I was also carrying on with plenty of normal parenting stuff: I gave a presentation in Nora's fifth-grade classroom (about what I have no recollection) the day after Brad went into the hospital. In the first couple of days, Brad FaceTimed with the kids, but as he got sicker and more disoriented that stopped. They wouldn't see him for nearly three months.

DAY ZERO

Like all hidden worlds, that of a bone marrow transplant has its own language. The day the transplant actually takes place is called Day Zero. In some transplant centers they call it the patient's second birthday. Brad's transplant was on a Monday night, and though his nurses told me it would be uneventful, even anticlimactic, I wanted to be there. They were right. Though a transplant sounds like a surgery, in this case the procedure is just cells dripping into an IV; it took place in his hospital bed, with me there in the room along with a watchful nurse and Dr. T. The main danger at the time of transplant is a potential allergic reaction, so Brad got a dose of Benadryl beforehand and dozed through much of the transfusion.

The bag of new stem cells from his brother was a surprising dusty-rose color, like a Laura Ashley dress from the '80s. Before the nurses hung it on Brad's IV tower—already teeming with saline and medications—they asked if I wanted to hold it. Sure, I said.

It was wobbly and heavy, like a water balloon. Its millions of cells were the only things between my husband and certain death. I held his life in my hand, an all-too-on-point manifestation of how I often felt as his caregiver. Soon enough the pink cells were snaking through the IV tube into him, over the fuzzy pale-blue robe I'd given Brad for Christmas. The medical team discussed the show dogs, basset hounds, belonging to one of the nurses. I tweeted a picture of that long, slender tubing full of pink cells. Eventually I went home, leaving the stuffiness of the hospital for the cool January night. The big event we had been waiting for had happened. Brad got the cells; no last-minute catastrophes had prevented it. Everything had gone smoothly. Now it was time to wait.

SUSPENDED IN ISOLATION

Locked away behind multiple sets of doors in a hospital tower, Brad was like a hairless Rapunzel, unreachable. His room in the BMTU had a small antechamber to protect him from the stray bacteria and viruses and fungi with which the hospital teemed. That little room was stocked with butter-yellow gauze gowns, all disposable; masks; gloves; hand sanitizer; a sink. The anticontagion precautions demanded we visitors wash our hands there and don a gown. At certain times, as when Brad had C. diff, we also had to wear gloves and masks. I never fully understood how it was determined that, say, the front of my clothes posed a risk but the bottom of my shoes didn't. Nothing about the way the isolation precautions functioned made sense to me; some of them seemed more like superstition than science. I later thought often of those masks and gowns, dozens a day just for Brad's room, during the coronavirus outbreak and its attendant mask shortages.

Of course, isolation—both medical, as in quarantines, and social or emotional—has always been a part of illness. Susan Sontag, writing more than forty years ago, when cancer was even more feared than it is now, points out that the isolation many ill people experience has a superstitious underpinning: "Any disease that is treated as a mystery and acutely enough feared will be felt to be morally, if not literally, contagious. Thus, a surprisingly large number of people with cancer find themselves being shunned by relatives and friends and are the object of practices of decontamination by members of their household, as if cancer, like TB, were an infectious disease. Contact with someone afflicted with a disease regarded as a mysterious malevolency inevitably feels like a trespass; worse, like the violation of a taboo."[2] Sontag's point stands even in a different era of cancer treatment: illness is a world apart, and by extension the world of caregiving is as well—with the added twist that caregivers may feel alienated from the loved one they're caring for, as I did.

In the wake of the transplant I visited Brad most days but I still felt like he was receding ever further from me. A calendar chart on his door tracked the days after transplant: +1, +2, and so on. His nurses marked any change in his white blood counts, which would be evidence of engraftment. Meanwhile, Brad was still struggling to eat. He resisted going on IV nutrition but when I saw his mouth was too sore to tolerate a milkshake, I pushed him even harder than his doctors were doing to shift to IV nutrition, called TPN. He, in pain and foggy from painkillers, was still putting updates on the blog we had started to keep friends and family informed about his status. The blog saved me the time and labor that would have been needed to update people individually and was invaluable in that way, but it also led to some dilemmas. Some family members didn't think we should be sharing so much information—and when I read Brad's rambling, painkiller-fueled entries, I started to see their point. As his entries started to get less coherent I wondered if I should cut him off from posting and whether I even had the right.

Slowly I learned the weird logic of the hospital. I knew where to cut through a stairwell for a shortcut to the elevators. I found out which kiosk had the best coffee and learned its hours so I never had to get coffee from the cafeteria. I roamed the halls to seek out odd and interesting art for a series I started posting on Instagram of #hospitalartdaily. I had some little social media lifelines, but in many ways I felt as isolated as Brad—though in a very different way. I felt like I was trapped forever in the in-between little room, an antechamber between the world of health and extreme sickness. I played Paul Simon's "Boy in the Bubble" often in those days—the age of miracles and wonders, but also of pain—and I thought I was playing it about Brad but maybe it was more about myself.

Nobody out in the regular world understood what the transplant entailed, and it was exhausting to try to explain. The only other time in my life that I've felt so set apart was during the early days of grief after my mother's death by suicide. It seemed incredible then that the world could be carrying on as normal, unaware of what had happened to her, to me.

During the most severe stages of Brad's illness I felt a comparable sense of grief. In the aftermath of the stem cell transplant, the partner I had was gone; he was replaced by someone unrecognizable. For many weeks he hovered a few notches below full consciousness. I could make little sense of what he said to me; he was sunk inward, with no ability to concentrate on anyone or anything else. Truth be told, that state persisted for years after the worst of his illness was over, and it still leaves its mark.

I felt a gulf not just between me and him but between me and the world. I was lonely—even though being alone, preferably with a book, used to be my favorite thing. I wasn't a confirmed loner as a kid, but I loved the retreat of reading, especially as a respite from my parents' fighting and my mother's volatile moods. When caregiving, the books I'd loved years before brought me a little bit of the same peace they had in childhood. In one, I rediscovered a dark story of caregiving in an unlikely place: L. M. Montgomery's Anne of Green Gables series, which I'd remembered mainly as sunny. But dark themes—the unhappiness of orphans, child mortality, rural poverty—creep around the edges of all the novels. The fifth book, *Anne's House of Dreams*, marks a radical departure from the bright world Anne usually inhabits.[3] In an odd, sensationalist subplot, Anne's new friend Leslie Moore becomes a caregiver for her brain-damaged husband. As a child I'd never considered Leslie's role in the narrative, as the dark shadow of Anne's happiness. But after Brad's diagnosis I often thought of the lessons it holds for modern caregivers like me. Leslie's plight seems insoluble, and therein, I argue, lies an example for the many of us who feel trapped in a life of caregiving. Caring for a very ill spouse has been for me, as it was for Leslie, a world apart. I, like her, have longed for a stormy night or a wild evening to slip out of the house and rage against fate.

Anne's House of Dreams opens with Anne marrying her true love, Gilbert Blythe. En route to their new house, Anne spots a stunningly beautiful woman in a white dress with a red flower, wandering the scenic Prince Edward Island shore with a flock of geese. The woman fixes the new bride with a baleful stare. Anne wonders about the beautiful girl for weeks. It turns out to be Leslie Moore, her reclusive neighbor. Leslie is twenty-eight but has been for twelve years a full-time caregiver for her husband, Dick, a onetime sailor and former abusive spouse. Leslie, raised in poverty, married him under duress at age sixteen. Dick soon after suffered a traumatic brain injury during a bar fight in Cuba, and is now—in the not-so-sympathetic phrasing of the community—an "imbecile" who requires constant care.

I can claim neither extraordinary beauty nor a flock of geese but I identify with that feeling of wandering the seashore, looking balefully on happiness. My husband also seems vastly different now from the man I married—though far less so than brain-injured Dick Moore. Like Leslie, I've learned the hard way that the experience of caregiving separates a person from friends, from family, even the ill person themself. Leslie's only defense, besides resentful staring, is her beauty: she maintains her "golden cloud" of hair at Crystal Gayle length and always makes sure she has a red accessory on somewhere, a flower or a ribbon. The gleam of color, Anne reflects at one point, expresses Leslie's personality, suppressed in her life of sorrow. It's a small but significant outlet, reminding me powerfully of the work of Ella Risbridger, who wrote for *The Pool UK* about caring for her partner through their stem cell transplant. She and I became friends via Twitter; her partner's course of treatment had many strange parallels with Brad's. Risbridger's recurrent theme was that keeping one's flame alive, in large part through things as simple as wearing a lipstick that makes you happy, is essential.[4] Before I ever read Risbridger's work I also made sure to have a gleam of red about me, like Leslie. I wore red lipstick to the hospital, even with yoga pants.

Leslie Moore's bitter expression of envy when she looks at Anne's happiness is one I often felt on my own face when I saw friends whose complacency or easy lives felt to me, in my frustration, almost offensive. When I reread *Anne's House of Dreams* as a caregiver, I wished for a narrative with Leslie, not Anne, as the protagonist, one with more of the daily details of her life. Montgomery is not much of a gritty realist, and she glosses kindly over backbreaking chores like laundry, the details of Dick's toileting and wound care, the tedium of entertaining a grown man with a toddler's capacities. We do get hints of Leslie's routines: the description of her "brown, work-hardened hands"; her mention of a day when "Dick had been very—very hard to manage"; her wondering aloud if she will follow her father to suicide as an escape.[5]

After settling in at Four Winds, Anne attempts to befriend Leslie, but there is a wide gulf between them, making the novel's examination of female friendship, as well as its twisting plot, more compelling than the earlier, simpler Green Gables books. Anne and Leslie have a friendship as rocky as the PEI shore they both wander. Anne can scarcely understand the difficulties between them; she is accustomed to everyone warming to her immediately, if not falling at her feet. But Anne, Leslie says, does not—cannot—understand her life's tragedy.

My situation as a caregiver and the fictional Leslie's were never equivalent; even when Brad was at his weakest, I had hope that he might continue to improve. So many caregivers, like Leslie, can look forward only to their charges' decline, or to long stasis—though it turns out that Leslie does escape, thanks to the magic of a rather far-fetched plot twist (see chapter 9). During the months of Brad's transplant and the longer years when he needed care, it wasn't just that I didn't have much time to see friends. I largely stopped getting invitations because people knew I was overwhelmed and didn't want to bother me. When I did socialize I couldn't relate to other people. I unfairly found their concerns trivial, so much so that I could hardly listen patiently; on the other hand, my problems were such a stone-cold bummer it really lowered the mood to talk about them. (Trust me; I have experience in bringing down a room. There's nothing like mentioning your mom's death by suicide to kill a conversation.) And I didn't want to talk about myself anyway. The challenge of explaining Brad's increasingly complex medical situation to people was beyond frustrating—not to mention how badly I wanted to scream at everyone who suggested he try turmeric or essential oils.

TAKE CARE, NOW

After Brad had been in the hospital for several weeks I was deep in the hospital routine. Visits usually began and ended with the parking garage, where the automated credit card machines were perpetually broken. Late afternoon usually found me in line after yet another long day of trying to track down doctors on rounds, attempting to escape so I could run an overdue errand (all hospitals should have mini Targets and maybe a bar), pick up our daughters from aftercare they didn't like, and get home. Even though I wished the automated machines worked to speed my departure, I appreciated the brief moment of human interaction with the parking-garage attendants. One in particular always offered a kind "You take care, now" after I paid. I liked hearing "take care" because it implicitly acknowledged things might be a little tough for the hospital-parking-garage crowd. At the time I never noticed the completely unintended double meaning of "take care," which could also be interpreted as a subtle imperative to do the thing I was already doing every day.

With apologies to Kelly Clarkson, what doesn't kill you sometimes beats you down, as was beautifully expressed in a moving poem by Suzanne Edison, first published in a 2018 special issue of the literary journal *Michigan Quarterly Review* devoted to caregiving. Edited by poet Heather

McHugh, the issue bears witness to the increasing cultural recognition of this mostly unseen labor. Edison's poem, "When My Child Fell Ill," critiques this cliché in its opening lines:

> *"what didn't kill me, left me*
> *Drained as bleached coral,*
> *Spongiform, a holy mess*
> *In unmapped reefs"*[6]

The ordeal of caregiving, Edison writes, "did not gift me a badge / or crown, did not ennoble."

In the same issue, Kim Wyatt writes in her essay "Terroir" of this feeling of being drained: "You don't really know how much caregiving will consume you."[7] Wyatt compares a drive in thick California fog to the feeling of caregiving: "What I like about the fog, even though I could drive into a ditch or a bay or a semi at any moment, is the metaphor: I can't see what lies ahead. I could conjecture all day long and it wouldn't mean a thing. . . . The advice I keep getting from people who have been caregivers to their parents is this: Do not plan too far ahead. The thing you think is going to happen will not be the thing that happens. I cling to this not-knowing like faith." The fogs she mentions aren't the high, scudding clouds of San Francisco, but thick ground fogs that rise up from the damp ground in the chilly, rainy winter season. Where I live in Sacramento, we call them tule fogs.[8] Here in the river bottom they are endemic and dangerous, especially on the road. Sometimes they are so thick I can't see across my own street. When I was a kid I loved them. Being in a warm house looking out at the fog felt like being wrapped in a duvet. I'm still fond of a foggy day but I also feel its hint of danger.

Not knowing what lies ahead, living with the dread of loss, unable to attend to one's basic needs because of the urgency of another person's: those are the aspects of caregiving that can't be conveyed by all the statistics in the world. I left the hospital each day in an exhausted mental fog so intense I sometimes could hardly figure out something as simple as how much money I needed to hand over for parking. "You take care, now," the parking-garage attendants sang out to me after such days, and I left with tears in my eyes. I needed every drop of kindness then.

GVHD

By Day +15, in late January, the calendar chart on Brad's isolation-room door was already reflecting engraftment and the transplant physicians were starting to talk about him going home. I was skeptical; it seemed far too fast. He was still suffering from C. diff and he wasn't eating much besides broth. And then, as we descended into the miserable month of February 2016, his hands started to itch and his stomach started to hurt.

Graft-versus-host disease (GvHD) is a confusing, uniquely modern ailment, like the inverse of rejection in a solid organ transplant. If you were to need and get a kidney donated from someone, for instance, there's a good chance your immune system would identify it as a foreign body and attack it. Thus, organ transplant recipients are given immune suppressants. In a stem cell (or bone marrow) transplant, sometimes the new immune system (the graft), in its unfamiliar environment, looks around and sees the entire body around it (the host) as foreign. It then, in unscientific terms, freaks the fuck out. GvHD can pop up in the liver, skin, gut, eyes, and plenty of other spots; its attacks, as with many autoimmune responses, often seem random.[9] The possibility of GvHD—which is termed "acute" when it arises within the first 100 days of transplant and "chronic" when it continues in the longer post-transplant period—is why stem cell transplant patients are kept on immunosuppressant medications even though the effectiveness of the transplant at fighting the cancer depends on the immune response. The medical team has a delicate balance to maintain: just enough immune response to keep the cancer from returning but not so much that GvHD gets out of control.

Brad, unlucky as usual, got it everywhere: gut, liver, skin, and eyes. First he had a stippled red rash on his skin and his hands swelled and peeled. But his doctors weren't convinced it was a GvHD response. He was furious at one of the doctors on the transplant team because of this, which gave me a challenging set of roles: advocating for him (I was pretty sure he was right about the GvHD) while also making peace with the doctor who had the power to order more treatment. It was only when the diarrhea began—and had to be measured by the quart—that the medical team was convinced enough to start the standard treatment of high-dose steroids.

The steroids at first had no effect. Diarrhea stripped his bowels and sloughed away blood and shit and cilia. He had Grade IV gastrointestinal

GvHD; IV is the worst grade (a key measure of the grades is the daily measurement of diarrhea, in quarts) and is fatal in most cases. His abdomen was distended, bloated with pain and IV fluids, and splotched with brilliant purple bruises from injections of blood thinners, administered to treat a blood clot. I wonder if the bruising became so severe in part because his subcutaneous architecture was so permanently altered. As the tumors shrank, had the new blood vessels that had grown to serve them remain? The cancer reshaped my husband's body, marking it with scars on and under the skin, with rashes, bruises, punctures, oozing blood, oozing shit, with constant pain. I didn't know if I would ever again lay my head on that small hollow below his left shoulder and idly rest my hand on his abdomen. I didn't know if I would want to.

It almost seemed like a cruel joke that 2016 was a leap year, adding an extra day to that terrible February. Brad's diarrhea was so severe that he sat on a commode most of the day (he could no longer walk the ten or so feet to his hospital room's bathroom), developing open sores on his elbows from leaning on the commode's rough plastic arms. The nurses wrapped towels around the plastic but these were even worse: hospital towels make sandpaper seem fluffy. Our daughter Nora, who was trying out sewing then, made some little pillows out of fleece printed with the logo of the San Francisco 49ers. The pillows helped his arms and they also helped give her a meaningful way to connect to the dad she couldn't see, to contribute to his treatment.

On one bad day I ran into his nurse coordinator from the Cancer Center in the elevator. I told her about how bad Brad seemed, and how much pain he was in, and how hard it was to watch. "The good news," she said with gentle compassion, "is that he won't remember much of it." She was right; he doesn't, at least not the worst of it. But I do. Part of the onus of caregiving is carrying memory.

At that time the nurses were managing most of Brad's physical care: changing IV bags, measuring diarrhea, getting him in and out of bed. My caregiving role seemed like it ought to be light but it didn't feel that way. I felt like a project manager trying to keep all the balls in the air. Just understanding his increasingly complicated case and translating it into lay terms to keep family and friends informed was a big job all on its own. Then there were matters of advocacy, of soothing Brad, and the smaller tasks like bringing the fresh socks and underwear he needed daily—a source of high anxiety for him.

The hardest for me, during the most intense flare of his GvHD, were the daily visits, something I increasingly came to dread. The room was hot, the visits moribund. I was impatient, always thinking of the things I needed to do. Brad couldn't engage with reports of the outside world or follow much conversation. One of his treatments—tincture of opium—was a surprising throwback, so his haze was understandable. He was often on the commode throughout the visit, diarrhea disgorging from him. Sitting by him was a kind of vicarious trauma.

LOVE AND DUTY

I'd have liked to think that love was going to get me through caring for Brad, but for me the motivation that really stuck was a sense of duty. I was so worn out and scared that my affection for my husband became tamped down, in what was probably a self-protective coping mechanism. What propelled me to go back to the hospital every day was the simple knowledge that I ought to—that I had promised to do so in our marriage vows and it was my duty to carry out that promise. That feeling, along with the tincture of opium, reminded me powerfully of the Victorian novels I'd studied and often returned to for pleasure. They are replete with laudanum, the bed-bound ill, the quietly suffering, the nervous invalids, and the angels in the house who dispense care and sympathy to all—while also, offstage, doing laundry, dressing bedsores, emptying bedpans, and concocting the jellied soups and delicate blancmanges that sustained the sick before hospital trays and packaged Jell-O. When Brad was able to try food again I imitated those women, simmering broths and carrying them hot to his bedside, hoping to coax my charge to take a few mouthfuls. As I imagine those women must have, I quelled an inner flare of resentment when most of the broth had to be discarded. All the care I poured into it couldn't guarantee he'd take in more than a spoonful.

The ties of duty might sound rather old-fashioned to modern ears but the literature of long ago is chock-full of such language—and caregivers. *Middlemarch*, my longtime favorite, includes a surprising amount of caregiving, which comes up—along with two sharp clashes between duty to the invalid and duty to self—in the novel's many interwoven plots.

Through its stories of caregiving, the novel grapples deeply with questions of women's love, women's duty, and the Venn diagram between the two. Nearly all middle-class women of the Victorian era—the primary audience for such novels—would have had painfully intimate experiences of caregiving. At that time, illness and death happened at home. Hospitals were places of horror, reserved for the indigent and quarantined. Though that shifted over the course of the nineteenth century as medicine became more professionalized, at the time *Middlemarch* was set, the 1830s, only the faintest stirrings of this change were apparent.[10]

The novel's heroine, the young, beautiful, idealistic Dorothea, has naively married the withered scholar Casaubon. His great project, a "Key to All Mythologies," turns out to be an antiquated boondoggle; the man, jealous and petty. Moreover, he suffers a heart ailment and becomes a semi-invalid when the marriage is already under severe strain. His doctor tells Dorothea—but not Casaubon—the diagnosis and says that he must rest. It is Dorothea's job to keep him from strain and work, a near-impossible task.

Medical ethics about patient consent have changed, and these days a doctor could not confide this sort of information to a spouse without telling the patient. And yet such dilemmas do arise: quandaries in which the caregiver must make decisions for a patient who is largely unaware, or who does not or cannot understand the danger to themself. When Brad was at his sickest—a time of which he now has only fragmentary memories—I looked up the mortality statistics for Grade IV GvHD. They were shocking: 90 percent. One day, when Dr. T and I were the only ones in Brad's room, with Brad himself in a semiconscious haze, I asked Dr. T about that. He was honest with me: there was, as my research suggested, an extremely high chance Brad wouldn't survive. I didn't share this with Brad until years later—at the time it seemed like it would cause him to lose hope. I didn't tell his parents either. Holding such knowledge on my own was a terrible trial. I understood all too well why after the doctor leaves that scene in *Middlemarch*, Dorothea bursts into tears.

ALIENATION THROUGH CARE

Part of the reason that my caregiving was fueled more by duty than by love was because Brad and I had become so alienated from each other, especially during his transplant. We were physically separated during his many hospitalizations, and when he was in isolation he was so ill and fragile we couldn't really touch, even to hold hands. The devastation that his illness unleashed on his body was terrible to witness. Brad was undergoing distress I couldn't imagine, even though I was there daily. My life outside the hospital became equally unintelligible to him. We couldn't even talk much about our daughters; he found it painful, and was often too removed from their concerns, and too heavily medicated, to engage. His world had shrunk to the confines of his hospital bed and nothing happening in the outside world held much interest. Even now I occasionally realize with a start that much of 2016 is a blank for him. I remember coming into the hospital room one day that February, after Beyoncé released "Formation," trying to tell him about it, and later playing *Lemonade* for him, to no interest. He missed the presidential primaries and debates too. I once mentioned the viral clip of Hillary and Bill Clinton gawking at the balloon drop at the Democratic Convention, only to remember he hadn't seen it.

When the glue of ordinary conversation and shared everyday experiences starts to crumble, it can be an effort to keep a relationship going. I knew I was withdrawing from Brad as he became sicker. To tell the truth, it was at least partly self-protective. I thought he was dying and I couldn't really bear to keep our bond as strong as it had been when losing him entirely seemed imminent.

Carrying on in the full awareness of that pain felt impossible. Instead, I had to care for him almost robotically, separating myself from my emotions. Sometimes, when the pain or indignity of his treatment was extreme, I almost had to pretend he was a stranger. Besides, I was so tired and there was so much to do. Pushing forward felt critical, as Abby Maslin describes in her memoir *Love You Hard*, her account of caring for her husband, TC, after he suffers a traumatic brain injury. When he is in the ICU, she must erase herself: "I must remain tethered to the present moment—disconnected from who I was yesterday and what I might become tomorrow. Not a mother. Not a teacher. Not even a wife. Until further notice, I am just a mass of energy burning through one minute and then the next."[11]

I worried—correctly—that the physical side of caregiving would damage our relationship. Maslin writes evocatively of feeling like she's intruding by caring for her husband: "Over the years, I've seen how this type of brutal intimacy has made it difficult for my parents, especially my mother, to return to the roles of husband and wife. If I see too much, will I begin to feel more like TC's nurse than I do his wife? Is this even a question caregivers are allowed to ponder? I've never known my husband's body like this. The mechanics of it. The excretions. The fluids."[12] Sometimes, in the hospital, I could see drops of shit on the floor or the sheets. I didn't want to cause Brad shame by telling him; his vision was so impaired he couldn't see the spots. But sometimes I had to take home soiled laundry, such as the light-blue robe he wore often in the hospital, or quietly throw out fouled underwear.

The up-close intimacies of caregiving are rarely publicly discussed but they can be an enormous challenge. Disgust, as my therapist told me recently, is a core emotion, and for caregivers dealing with feces or vomit or wound care—especially those of us without medical training or the inclination toward it—it may be natural to feel squeamish, horrified, or alienated from the care recipient. That's no less true for adult children caring for parents than it is for spouses like me, though the underlying emotions may be different. Such feelings are often accompanied by other emotions: guilt for the caregivers, shame for the care recipients. Both can be corrosive to the original bond. Still, at least for me, the challenge of the physical relationship of caregiving was more straightforward than its emotional entanglements and clashes of judgment.

Often, Brad's perspectives were at direct odds with mine. One such time came a couple of months after his transplant, when his chimerization—the proportion of his blood cells now carrying his brother's DNA rather than his own—was tested. (A chimera, scientifically and medically speaking, is an organism containing two types of genetic material. Post-transplant, if the graft succeeds, patients have both their own and their donors' DNA in perpetuity.) The various numbers from Brad's routine daily blood draws weren't looking good and the doctors were worried the graft might be failing—which could be fatal or could necessitate a second transfusion of stem cells, itself a risky move that could trigger more GvHD. The test, however, found that 100 percent of Brad's cells bore his brother's genetic signature, meaning the graft was holding—unquestionably good news. One of the charge nurses—the term for nurse supervisors who manage schedules and other supervisory tasks, and with whom we had frequent contact over the years of Brad's treatment—had become buddies with Brad. That nurse got carried away and burst into his room saying, "Good news, man! The test came back! You beat cancer!"

Brad was elated. When my in-laws, who had been present, told me what had happened, I was enraged. The chimerization test, as the doctors had explained it to me, indicated no such thing. Brad remained very sick and at high risk of death from the complications of transplant. In most stem cell transplants of the type Brad had, the doctors do not expect or test for any return of cancer until at least three months post-cancer. And even a scan at that time is far from definitive: a relapse, though most likely in the first year post-transplant, could occur at any time.

In one way there was really no reason for me to be so furious; it didn't hurt Brad to have a little hope. But my head was a constant whirl of emotion and logistics then. I was worried about false hope and fallout and the setbacks that always seemed to be lurking around the next bend. I was working so hard, then, to stay on an even keel.

THREE

ON HIS BLINDNESS

BMTU, Part Two

Shortly after his GvHD onset, Brad began to feel excruciating eye pain. At first the medical team was baffled, thinking it was pinkeye or another infection. Chronic ocular GvHD is common enough, usually taking the form of discomfort or dry eyes, but an acute flare-up immediately after transplant is extraordinarily rare. By the time Brad's doctors recognized the eye irritation and burning pain for what it was, the inflammation had scarred his corneas—something no medical personnel on his unit had ever before seen. His corneas, normally clear hard shields over the lens, were so scarred that, like a glass window scratched by a diamond, they obscured his vision. At first this cloudy effect made it increasingly hard for him to read or recognize people; at the worst of his visual impairment he could see only whether it was light or dark—there was little else than a vague blur. After three years of fluctuating vision and four eye surgeries, he recovered nearly full sight. But when that first eye pain struck, and as his visual acuity plummeted, everything was uncertain.

The hospital seemed to have no idea what to do—hardly anyone suddenly goes blind once they're already admitted. It had never happened before on the bone marrow transplant unit; they barely even knew how to reach Ophthalmology. Once they did, it was hard to get the ophthalmology team to Brad's bedside. They were an entirely outpatient service, in clinic during regular business hours, unaccustomed to making hospital rounds.

TO BE EYES AND HANDS TO YOU

Brad's eye injury was something only advanced medical science could have produced, yet it reminded me sharply of the later chapters of *Jane Eyre*, when Jane flees Rochester's Thornfield Hall to be her own mistress after she learns he is already married—but then returns to him to become his caregiver. Rochester has been blinded in a fire set by his mad first wife, Bertha Mason Rochester, which destroys Thornfield Hall; in despair he calls out to Jane, who is mysteriously able to hear him from a long distance away. When she returns to him she pledges to serve as both his eyes and hands, his nurse and housekeeper. Patient Jane becomes the good caregiver of the novel named for her, the selfless opposite of Bertha's drunken, inattentive caregiver, Grace Poole. Jane is willing, she says, to become his eyes—to sacrifice all she might wish to see in order to privilege his vision—and she is willing to do this whether they marry or not.

Reader, as we all know, Jane married him. When she accepts him she tells him, "I love you better now, when I can really be useful to you, than I did in your state of proud independence."[1] If this is the test of a good helpmeet—or was in the nineteenth century—I failed it when Brad, too, went blind. One challenge of caregiving in our modern marriage was for us to find a path through Brad's blindness together, and to reframe our ways of seeing each other through a loss we'd never expected. This raised painful questions about both the nature of our marriage and how I could best care for him without losing myself.

I thought often of Jane extending her hand to Rochester as I chafed against Brad's new dependency. It was particularly painful that he could no longer read and write—both crucial to his and my self-conception. Like Rochester, he was never completely blind. Rochester can see the faint glow of the fireplace, a luminous halo around candlelight, with one of his eyes, promising some form of reprieve. Brad, too, could see blurry shapes.

Until Brad lost his sight, I never noticed how pervasive metaphors of vision are in everyday speech. See you later. It's nice to see you. The way I see it. A new vision for the future. Can you take a look at this? I don't know, but we'll see. Let's look it up. I'll watch for your message. I'll keep an eye on it. Look, I'm trying to explain. Do you see? And then someone I love went blind and suddenly I saw (see what I mean?) my casual "Okay then, I'll see you later" in a whole new light. Because that person, visionless, would not be seeing me. But I did see him, always.

My vision became merciless as Brad's clouded. I saw things I would wish on nobody: his oncologist's hopeless grim look, dire statistics on GvHD mortality in medical studies, eggplant-purple bruises on his tortured abdomen, our daughters crying, puffy dark bags under my tired eyes. I saw the world, the blue sky, the snowcapped Sierra Nevada mountains from his eighth-floor isolation room. I saw trees below leaf out and flowers bloom and evenings lengthen as January, when he entered the hospital, gave way to February, when he almost died, and in turn March and April and May.

During those months I felt literally and figuratively unseen by Brad and many others, as our former lives dissolved like a movie shot into his urgent struggle for survival, me blurred in the background. None of us could see the future: the most advanced scan couldn't reveal whether cancer cells might regrow and no instrument could peer below opaque corneas.

Brad's blindness was uncertain, frustrating. The eye team, none of whom had seen ocular GvHD before, could not offer a clear prognosis or predict whether the condition would heal. They continued to appear at odd moments; their arrival in Brad's isolation room was always an event, reminding me of the "eminent oculist" from London who pronounces on Rochester's vision.[2] The most eminent oculist of all, however, a courtly specialist, could not come to Brad's bedside. He didn't have hospital privileges, which meant that Brad had to go to him, despite his fragility. Moving Brad involved dressing him in full protective gear (gown, booties, hat, gloves, N95 mask) and putting him on a stretcher for transport by ambulance to a building down the block from the hospital. I was waiting at the outpatient clinic and I saw the eyes of all the waiting patients widen when Brad was wheeled in. I knew, of course, that he looked deathly ill, but seeing others see him was an extra jolt of reality.

As Brad's vision worsened, that most eminent oculist decided on a tarsorrhaphy, a word I had to look up. I quelled a full-body shudder when I learned it involved sewing his eyes shut. The medical reasoning was that constant, involuntary blinking over dry, inflamed eyes was aggravating the corneal scratches and not allowing them to heal; keeping the eyes shut and lubricated might promote recovery. Cross my heart, hope to die, stick a needle in my eye: I am not squeamish about much, but I abhorred the thought of that fine needle passing through his eyelids. So did Brad, and I held his hand to steady us both, looking away as a nervous young resident thrust the needle beneath stubby lashes. Afterward, an inverted V of fine drawstrings was stuck to Brad's forehead, like exaggerated eyebrows. His nurses had to use the strings to lever open his eyelids, like Venetian blinds, to administer drops. His patience with that fussy, four-times-daily procedure and long days in isolation astonished me.

WHO ONLY STAND AND WAIT

When Brad couldn't see well enough to read, people often asked me if he was bored. It was a natural question—Brad had been an English professor, a writer, and an avid reader before his illness—and it saddened me to say no. His health was too poor to permit the focus or the drive to miss reading or writing.

In those days, when I frequently spent hours sitting in Brad's hospital room with little to do, I thought often of the well-known final line of John Milton's sonnet "On His Blindness": "They also serve who only stand and wait." When I went to look up the whole sonnet I was surprised by its relevance to Brad's situation. In it, the devout Puritan poet wrestles with the ramifications for his work of his fading vision—possibly the result of bilateral retinal detachment—which left him completely blind by the age of forty-three, in 1652. He would browbeat his daughters into serving as amanuenses and go on to compose his most famous work, *Paradise Lost*, after losing his sight. In this earlier sonnet, however, he laments his loss, meditating on how best to serve God when "that one talent which is death to hide," his writing, is "lodg'd with me useless."

Milton begins the sonnet worrying he is not resigned enough to God's will, saying that those "who best/ Bear [God's] milde yoke, they serve him best."[3] By the time he reaches that famous final line, however, he has found a measure of peace with his less active role in the world. The sonnet's resolution reminded me of Brad, bearing the hospital regimen. The hospital makes people patients; it also makes them patient. Every tiny action of its vast bureaucratic machine trains its denizens to wait, and its not-so-mild yoke fostered in Brad Miltonian patience.

Brad's patience may have served his cause better than I did. I struggled against the hospital's smooth slow logic; though I tried to remind myself I also served by standing (or, more usually, sitting) and waiting, I was thinking all the time of everything I'd left undone. Unlike Jane Eyre, I never found joy in subsuming myself. I demanded, I begged nurses for action, I invaded the room where the hospital fellows were at work to ask for updates. But I probably did Brad the most good when I simply sat and held his hand. On one visit our conversation turned especially serious as we looked ahead (there's that vision metaphor again) to our future. The doctors no longer thought Brad would die, but of his likely future quality of life or whether he would regain his sight they could tell us little.

"I don't understand why you're not excited about the future," Brad said. "I've made it."

I looked around his hospital room. Bags of yellow nutritional formula and dozens of medications hung on his IV tower, dripping into two chest catheters beneath his scratchy green gown. I gazed at the sewn-shut lids of eyes once blue as the sky.

"I don't understand why you *are* excited," I said. "What do you see in our future?"

"I'll get better," he said. "I'll regain my vision and strength and we'll travel and do all the things we always wanted to. This is for you. I'm getting better for us. Can't you see that?"

I paused. "That's the best possible outcome. But there are so many others. Ones where your vision doesn't recover, where your body doesn't recover, where you have chronic GvHD. Or where you relapse. I hope your vision is the right one. But I feel like we have to be prepared for others."

We fell into glum silence that, after a long pause, turned to honest communication about our fears. We hadn't talked like this, like spouses, for weeks; Brad had been too sick and I too walled off. In our conversation I said the word we had all been avoiding: "blind." We talked in real terms about what it might mean if he were to be sightless permanently, a prospect that terrified him. Losing his vision, I said, would not mean the loss of his essential self. He could still connect with words, with language, with poetry. He could adapt. Life might not match the rosy vision of the future that he held but it could still be more than worthwhile.

"You will not lose who you are," I said. "You may be blind. You may. But there are ways to get around this. You will still be you."

He cried.

"Look at Milton," I said. "He wrote, and he had fewer options for help than you do."

"I'm not Milton," he said.

"Maybe not. But you're a poet, and you can and will keep writing, even if it's hard."

We lacked the faith that had sustained Milton; Brad's religion, if anything, has always been literature. It was that he wished to serve, and I knew he needed to hear that his vision loss wouldn't mean the end of his writing. Through all the barriers that his cancer built between us, every so often came these sharp reminders: married nearly two decades, we knew each other inside and out.

"You can learn Braille and technological adaptations. You can listen to audiobooks and have an amanuensis. Remember when I read to Ved Mehta and helped with his edits? There's some grad student out there who can do that for you."

Mehta, blind since childhood, formerly wrote for the *New Yorker*. When I was in graduate school he had a visiting appointment at my university and I worked for him as an amanuensis. I never thought much about what his wife was doing with her time. Later, when Brad came home from the hospital, we hired a grad student to do the same tasks for him. Did she wonder what I was up to instead of reading to my husband? I couldn't bear the thought of subsuming my work to his even more than I already had. Navigating our marriage and our separate identities in the face of this new disability challenged us as it did not change the selfless Jane Eyre, who rhapsodizes at one point about how she never wearies of being Rochester's eyes.

That night in the hospital, all this lay in the future. I reassured him: "You'll learn. And I'll be there to help you. You'll write, even if you are blind."

Brad thanked me for saying the word "blind" aloud. What he needed then more than possibly empty reassurances that his vision would return was the knowledge that he—we—would cope if it didn't.

ON NOT COPING

Privately, though, I wasn't so sure I could cope. The faux-upbeat quasi-realism I employed in our blog was spilling into my relationship with my husband. I felt like a shell of a person—like a robot, carrying out my duty most of the time, unable to feel much as I did it. The peculiar feeling of alienation was heightened by having others around me nearly all the time, even at home, but not feeling that I could confide in any of them. My spouse, once the foundation of my support system, was the sick one and I was meant to be strong for him. I've long been a convert to the "ring theory" of grief, which—as explained in a viral *Los Angeles Times* article from 2013 called, bluntly, "How Not to Say the Wrong Thing"—advises you to imagine people in a stressful situation as occupying a series of concentric circles, with those most deeply affected in the center, and to "comfort in, dump out."[4] I wasn't exactly sure where to dump. Our rings felt warped somehow, like I was some kind of bump, or maybe an invisible layer. It was especially hard, then, living in the middle of a multigenerational household with my in-laws. Lucy was acting out a lot in her dad's absence (not surprisingly), and parenting with an audience didn't help. At the same time it was hard to witness the closed circle of a mutually supportive marriage while that relationship was missing for me.

Brad had been broken down to an almost infantile state of dependency: incontinent, unable to walk or feed himself, reliant on nurses. It was hard to watch this happen to my husband and hard to assume the quasi-parental, cheerleading role needed to take on to push him through his anxiety toward recovery. Even years later he still needs the occasional push, and it's a source of conflict for us. This nurse-patient dynamic felt, I think, more alienating to me than it did to Brad's parents, who, after all, first experienced him as their dependent.

Mostly I was able to do a reasonable imitation of a person who was coping, but sometimes the façade cracked. I tried my best to hold it together when I was around other people, and it felt like I was always around other people for whom I needed to put on a good face. Sometimes I screamed out loud in the car between the hospital and picking up the kids from aftercare, which they complained about often. Sometimes I drank a little too much bourbon after the girls were in bed and cried alone in my room.

One day in the hospital, though, the façade cracked in two. I was posting frequent updates on our blog, trying to translate Brad's complicated situation into something concerned friends would understand. In one March entry I'd said something about the stem cells from James causing Brad's GvHD, which I saw as simple fact. Brad's mom, however, read it as a hurtful insult to James and worried that he, too, would read it amiss. I can't remember who told me she was upset: maybe Brad or maybe a nurse. Whatever happened, even that mild, secondhand criticism sent me into full meltdown. I ran out of the stuffy hospital room, into the hall, to cry—for which read "sob out loud"—in the hall. I couldn't stop. I knew patients couldn't hear me, since all the rooms on the BMTU had double doors, and I almost never saw another family member on the unit. But I was plainly unnerving the nurses. It didn't matter; I couldn't stop. Brad's nurse followed me and steered me into a tiny room I'd never seen before. A secret crying room! Who knew? I might have taken advantage of it a lot sooner if I had. I hadn't cried much in the weeks just after the onset of Brad's GvHD, when I thought he was dying. I couldn't spare the emotional energy. But as he improved a little I had some space to give in to my feelings, much as Leslie does one day in *Anne's House of Dreams* when Anne finds her friend "weeping horribly—with low, fierce, choking sobs, as if some agony in her soul were trying to tear itself out." Anne leaves, understanding Leslie might never forgive a friend who found her in her "abandonment of despair."[5] I've always had a hard time forgiving those who see my despair too. Given the choice I'll do my crying in a little room, one with a door. Like Leslie Moore I was proud, and growing up with a difficult mother I'd learned that vulnerability didn't serve me well. I felt, as another character says of Leslie, like underneath my defenses my soul must be raw. Sometimes my isolation was self-imposed because I couldn't stand having that rawness touched. I couldn't take anyone's pity; I felt I could hold it together only as long as I wasn't being scrutinized. And yet, like Leslie Moore, I was painfully lonely and needed support. I'm not sure how long I sobbed but I do know the nurse had to go for an extra box of tissues.

OUT OF THE ATTIC

Back at home, it was when a dead bat fell out of the ceiling that I thought I might really lose it. It lay, angular gray limbs curled, on the second step down of our wide stairs. Six feet from my younger daughter's bedroom. Ten feet from mine. The girls were in the bath: "Stay there," I yelled. The bat had definitely not been on the stairs five minutes before, when we had come upstairs for their baths. I looked up at the ceiling. It was April, the first summer-warm night of the year, and I'd turned on the whole-house fan in an attempt to cool off the hot upstairs. The dead bat—at least it was dead—must have fallen from the wide slats of the vent.

I'd just taken the girls to an art therapy group for kids affected by cancer. It meant coming home a little late and bundling the wound-up kids into bed. I was tired and on edge, worried by rumblings from Brad's doctors that they might send him home soon.

It had been my bright idea to install the whole-house fan. It works well in Sacramento, where summer days are hot—often above 100 degrees Fahrenheit—but nights can cool off by 40 degrees or so. The whole-house fan vents through the attic and sucks cool air from outside into the entire house when you open a few windows downstairs. It turned out that dust and other detritus had collected on the wide slats over the winter. In this case, detritus is a nice word for "mummified bat."

So, we had bats in the attic. Shit. If Brad came home he would be on immunosuppressants. What diseases did bats have? Rabies? How many of them were up there? How long had this one been there? Long enough to die and dry out, obviously. What else might be lurking in the attic? How the hell was I going to get rid of this disgusting fucking bat when I couldn't bear to even walk past it? The rational part of my brain knew this tiny, extremely deceased mammal couldn't hurt me, but my body recoiled at approaching it, much less touching it. I told the girls about the bat, and they shrieked.

I would love to be someone who can calmly dispose of a dead bat, but I wasn't a great feminist role model that night. My overwhelming reaction was, fuck all this noise. It was like a twist on the Talking Heads song: not my beautiful house, not my beautiful life. In the life I had built, the life I was living before cancer so rudely interrupted, my husband was there in part to pick up the goddamn bat. If he teased me a little bit about not wanting to pick up various dead vermin, I didn't resent it because I knew he didn't think any less of me. A dead bat on my stairs wasn't the biggest crisis compared to cancer and nearly dying. But it was an immediate one, and that bat wasn't going away by itself.

In the end my father-in-law got rid of the bat, and the girls calmed down enough to go to sleep (in my room), and the next day I called some bat-control specialists. I learned a lot about bat removal. The first thing: it is very expensive to get bats out of your attic, and it doesn't matter whether you are removing a huge colony or just a few bats. (We had the latter.) To get them out you have to seal every single crack in your entire house larger than a quarter inch, and then the exterminator installs one-way exits. So at night, when the bats go out to hunt insects, they can't come back in. It takes a few weeks. It was good I had called when I did, the bat specialist told me. Pupping season was coming up and you can't get rid of them during it. Okay, I said, wondering why baby bats are called pups. Then he told me how to recognize bat guano. You can tell it's bat guano, he said, because if you crush the little piece it disintegrates into powder, which rat shit doesn't do.

I joked that maybe the guano was worth something. After all, guano is used for fertilizer—there was even a nineteenth-century guano rush on some small islands near Peru. Could that offset the cost, maybe? He didn't think that was funny. So I paid the money (it came to about $250 per suspected bat), got the house sealed up tightly, and waited for the bats to leave.

That hot April night the bat was the least of what came out of the attic—though I can still picture it curled there, like a tiny gray demon at the top of our wide staircase. That one tiny mummy bore a ridiculous symbolic weight. Somehow the dead bat, the dust, the crumbly guano, felt like the perfect symbol of all the rage and resentment I'd been hiding away. It made me feel, well, batshit crazy, like every cliché of female madness out there. Summer was coming, with its heat; Brad was recovering, bit by tiny bit. Soon he'd be coming home to a house that might be full of bats, to rabies and madness, to my wavering sanity. Like the bat, I wanted out of the attic; like another madwoman before me, the reason I wanted to escape my attic was to set fire to my no longer beautiful life. As a baby Victorianist in the take-back-the-night 1990s, I cut my teeth on Sandra Gilbert and Susan Gubar's *The Madwoman in the Attic*, a foundational feminist critical work that in part looks at Bertha Mason as a symbol of repressed female rage.[6]

Gilbert and Gubar's argument might seem obvious now, after intervening decades of feminist literary criticism, but when it appeared it was groundbreaking: Bertha Mason and Jane Eyre represent the dichotomy of the Victorian feminine, stripped down to its essentialist, patriarchal form: monstrous madwoman on the one hand, angel in the house on the other. Bertha Mason is the grotesque, angry, raging side of the female; Jane learns to tamp down her righteous anger and moments of rebellion as a child, and as an adult exercises utter self-control.[7] More broadly, Gilbert and Gubar contend that the woman writer of the day, too, was limited to this false dichotomy, lending a story like *Jane Eyre* a feminist subtext. In the novel, of course, it's a failure of caregiving that lets Bertha loose to burn things down. I felt like the mad wife and the failed caretaker, all rolled into one.

DISCHARGE

The possibility of Brad coming home became ever more real as April turned to May. As tired as we all were of the hospital, his care needs were overwhelming. He was still visually impaired and his tarsorrhaphy, which required a good two hours of hands-on care per day, was still in place. (In the end, it was taken out before he was discharged but he was still functionally sightless.) He was on intravenous nutrition for ten hours a day. He couldn't walk, shower, use the toilet, or dress independently, much less prepare food for himself. His hands shook with tremors from neuropathy. I was shocked to learn what kinds of care I was expected to administer, just as I had been the year before when Brad went home on IV antibiotics.

Because Brad's needs at home would be so complicated, I asked to meet with his entire care team in what was called a discharge conference. The idea was to discuss in detail his needs and how to manage them. I came with an extra advocate, a friend who was launching a business as a care coordinator. We were her guinea-pig clients and she was invaluable during the discharge process, especially in advising what I should be asking for. But asking the right questions didn't always help. At one point in the conference a particularly callous senior physician waved aside my concerns about administering intravenous nutrition, saying that patients could "just plug it in." She seemed to mean that a patient could self-administer the nutrition even without a caregiver's assistance, which would be possible in some cases but certainly not in Brad's. The process, far from an easy plug-in, was a complex, multistep procedure involving delicate operations such as using a syringe to inject a vitamin pack into the bag of TPN and slowly priming the pump before attaching it to an external catheter. Just setting it up took a minimum of twenty minutes, and that was after I got good at it.

We had a dedicated caseworker at Brad's health insurance company, who called me to say she felt he still had too many complications and would be safer, for now, in the hospital. It struck me as telling that even the insurance company would rather pay for him to stay in the hospital than send him home. But the hospital insisted. I've long suspected—though I can't be sure—that Brad was discharged when he was partly because he was nearing the end of the contracted length of stay negotiated for stem cell transplant patients. By discharging him, over my protests, the medical group transferred the responsibility for excess costs—including the hidden opportunity costs associated with the time it took me to coordinate care, negotiate with insurance, and care for Brad myself—directly to us.

At first I asked whether it might not be better to send him to a skilled nursing facility for more rehab, but that insurance caseworker went to bat for us to get comprehensive in-home rehab services covered, a rarity. Even she, however, couldn't get coverage for home-care workers, who are never covered by insurance. The hospital discharge coordinators were practically throwing equipment at us too: A wheelchair! A bigger pill organizer! A commode! A shower chair! Did he need a walker? (I had no idea, but he declined. He accepted a cane, though, and he already had a white cane for visual impairment.) Did he need grab bars in the shower and by the toilet? (Yes; the discharge department referred me to an installer.) Meanwhile I was deep-cleaning the house, getting the exterior washed, having the car detailed: everything had to be as sanitary as possible.

In the lead-up to discharge, Dr. T told me that after Brad came home he would need attendance twenty-four hours a day and could not be left alone even for a moment. When I pointed out that I had two children and they needed to be taken places, such as school, he replied, "Well, usually family steps in and it works out fine."

I wanted to ask the doctor whether his family was available, because mine certainly wasn't. My father and brother live ninety minutes away. By the time of Brad's discharge my in-laws had already been in California to help for more than four months. The assumption that all patients have care help standing by is common, as memoirist Anne Boyer—who was discharged over her own protests the same day she had a double mastectomy—notes: "You are not supposed to be alone when you get home. . . . But no one really asks how you manage it once you are forced out of the surgical center—who, if anyone, you have to care for you, what sacrifices these caregivers might have to make or the support they require."[8]

I got the distinct feeling that speaking up about the hardship of providing twenty-four-hour care was considered in poor taste—a caregiving faux pas, a sign I was insufficiently committed to my husband's recovery. Everyone involved with his discharge clearly preferred not to know how we would manage. It was as if it had been rendered invisible by the Somebody Else's Problem Field in Douglas Adams's *The Hitchhiker's Guide to the Galaxy*. I was not a person to them; I was an element of their patient's treatment.

With the help of my care-coordinator friend, I spent the days leading up to discharge frantically interviewing and hiring attendants who could be at our house twenty-four hours a day. The coordinator helped slow down the discharge process a little but I was still not ready when, on May 10, the hospital announced that the next day would be it. Brad would be coming home.

That sounded like, and was, an occasion to celebrate for our family. I tried to seem calm and even happy but I was overwhelmed with fears. That night I couldn't sleep. I was terrified and alone. It was 11 p.m., and most people I know go to bed early. I tried texting my brother, the only person I could think of who might be up, to see if he could talk, but there was no reply.

I needed a human connection of some kind in order to face the next frightening day, which felt like a closing trap. So I called a suicide hotline—the thing we tell all people experiencing despair to do. There's help out there, we're assured. I called, nervous. The voice at the other end of the hotline asked if I was actively suicidal. I said I wasn't planning anything right then but I was in despair. She asked if she could place me on hold to continue talking with someone in more serious crisis. I thanked her and hung up.

In the world of triage that hotline worker was right to talk to the person with active suicidal impulses. But I did wonder why there wasn't a hotline to help the people who are in a crisis a notch lower. (Since then, the Caregiver Action Network has launched a hotline for caregivers, called the Caregiver Help Desk, at 855-227-3640.[9]) After calling, I felt even more trapped and alone than before. After a night of poor sleep I took the girls to school, tidied up, and then went to the hospital to bring home my profoundly ill husband. What I didn't know then, but sensed, was that everything was about to get worse.

FOUR

CAREWORN

Life After Discharge

As I drove Brad home from the hospital I thought about two other trips home we'd made from the same hospital six and ten years before, with our babies. Then, I was the one with halting, weak steps while Brad proudly carried the baby in the car seat. I sat in the back, nervous and overwhelmed. But I was twice as worried now and Brad was the one unnerved by the expanse of the world. He couldn't see much beyond the brightness of the light but he could feel the motion of the car.

My feelings about Brad's homecoming were as mixed as they'd ever been. Certainly I was glad to be done with daily trips to the hospital, and we had our moments of exhilaration and laughter. When Dr. T, signing the discharge papers, said, "Do you realize you've been here 129 days?" Brad snapped back, with a flash of his old humor, "Nobody keeps me in the hospital 130 days!" But there were so many things to do, so many obstacles to living our lives, so many complications and considerations that couldn't be understood by the friends responding to the news with a quick "Woo-hoo! Great news!" comment on Facebook.

For starters there was the simple question of how to get him into the house. There was no easy way. Like many Sacramento homes ours is what's called a high-water bungalow, built four or so feet off the ground to accommodate the periodic floods that used to take place regularly before the days of regional flood control. All the entrances have steps and Brad was so weak that climbing even a single stair was an extreme challenge. I decided we'd go in through the only ground-level door, though that led to a landing between the main floor and basement—a potential plummet for someone uncertain of their balance. It had a high threshold that Brad would have to step over and several steps either up or down.

Our house has three levels (four if you count the onetime bat-infested attic): upstairs, with bedrooms; the elevated main floor; and a finished basement, which has a guest room. Brad had slept in the basement room when he'd come home from the hospital a year before, weakened and on oxygen. Now he would sleep there again. It had its own bathroom (now with grab bars installed) and fewer fall risks than our upstairs. Downstairs also had a TV and a big comfortable couch for the home-care workers I'd hired, who would be there round the clock. The IV tower was ready to house Brad's heavy bags of IV nutrition and a commode was set up. Brad had refused a hospital bed and I couldn't say I blamed him, but I worried about the bed we did have, which was high off the floor and had no place to grab if Brad needed to pull himself up to stand. Well, I consoled myself, that was why I'd hired home care.

The mile drive home from the hospital went by quickly, my thoughts whirling all the way. I turned the car sharply at the end of our long driveway and pulled up as close to the lemon trees as I could, underneath our back deck. The disadvantage of parking here was that the old brick and concrete paving was uneven, the footing treacherous. The advantage was that it was as close as possible to that side door.

Getting Brad out of the car took strength: I offered a hand, he leaned hard, and I pulled. His walk was a slow, slow shuffle. I warned him of the uneven pavement, the loose bricks. Step by agonized step we made our way to the side door. His foot caught on the high door frame as he tried to step up. He made it and there was a pause on the landing. My mother-in-law, waiting for us, stood above him, and I below, as he made his way up the stairs to the living room. It seemed to take hours. We led him to the couch. I have a picture of him lying there, that first day, pallid and exhausted. I was tired too, not from the physical effort as he was but from the mental and emotional strain of coordinating this homecoming. He fell asleep. I started a load of laundry and then I sat down and began organizing his thirty-five prescriptions according to the complex chart from the hospital pharmacist.

CARE WORK

Our home-care workers, Nancy and Emali, started the day Brad came home. They each worked a twelve-hour shift (Emali in the day, Nancy at night), which I knew was sure to be hard on them. I remember timidly asking, when interviewing them, whether we could use three shift workers for eight hours each—a more humane schedule, though maybe more challenging to manage. They firmly said they preferred the longer ones. I paid them directly, $15 per hour, each week—above minimum wage but nowhere near as much as their work was worth. Larger agencies, from which I also considered hiring, charged closer to $25 per hour but the actual attendants netted less than that.

Nancy ran a small, family-based home-care agency. She and Emali, and all their family, are Fijian. In our part of California, Fijians and Filipinos—some immigrants, others American born—dominate home caregiving work. As Ai-jen Poo notes in *The Age of Dignity*, "Immigration issues are inseparable from the issue of caregiving . . . two-thirds of nannies, housekeepers, and caregivers for the elderly are foreign-born."[1] This makes professional caregivers highly vulnerable to exploitation. According to Poo, caregivers earn on average less than $10 per hour—well below a living wage and below the minimum wage in many states[2]—and few receive sick or vacation days or other benefits. Poo notes professional caregivers suffer high rates of injury and burnout; few ever receive severance or notice when they are terminated.[3] (Often, professional caregivers' jobs end abruptly when a care recipient dies.) All care and domestic workers are vulnerable to being cheated out of wages, and because many of them are undocumented workers they have little recourse in labor disputes. All of these factors lead to an undervaluing of care in a society that doesn't consider it "real" work and has systematically stripped it of not only economic value but also of dignity.

In hiring Nancy and Emali, I participated directly in the common scenario for care in the United States: a white woman delegating, at relatively low wages, the care of a loved one to women of color. That's a longstanding and problematic pattern, one replicated across all of the care-based professions, including childcare and eldercare.

According to a 2014 fact sheet from PHI (formerly known as Paraprofessional Healthcare Institute), a nonprofit advocacy group working to improve the direct-care sector, 91 percent of home-care workers are female, 56 percent are nonwhite, 24 percent are foreign born, and 21 percent are single parents. Home-care aides earn near poverty wages, with a median hourly wage of less than $10 per hour.[4] Historically, most paid care workers operating in a domestic setting—even those employed by home-care agencies—have been excluded from labor protections in the United States, such as those provided by the Fair Labor Standards Act. Isolated within their work environments, lacking both legal protections and benefits, they are uniquely vulnerable to abuse.[5] While paid care workers are not the direct subject of this book, any consideration of family caregiving must reckon with the spillover effect of outsourcing care: the net effect is often the further exploitation of nonwhite workers. In other words, increased freedom from caring for the (predominantly white) group of privileged, unpaid family caregivers results in less freedom and more low-wage jobs for some of the least privileged women in the workforce. Approximately one in three unpaid caregivers uses paid services to help care for a loved one.[6]

Nancy and Emali relieved me of many hands-on tasks like laundry, food preparation, and administering Brad's eye drops and medications. They helped Brad get dressed, stand up out of bed, shower, and get to and from the bathroom or commode. They also cleaned and disinfected the commode, something I had a hard time bringing myself to do. I'd already seen too much of what my husband's body had gone through in the hospital and I worried our relationship had tipped irretrievably into a caregiver-patient one. Having care workers to handle the more physical aspects of caring felt like a small step toward normalcy.

Eventually, Emali began taking Brad to a few of his routine appointments. For instance, every other week he had to go to the hospital for two consecutive days for outpatient photopheresis, which took three to five hours and was located in a wing of the hospital far from the parking garage. Brad, unable to walk long distances, used a wheelchair, which added to the logistical challenge. Emali's work saved me hours on each of those days. Similarly, I taught Nancy to hook up the TPN nightly and disconnect it in the morning, which allowed me to get more rest and eventually spend time away from home. Nancy slept part of the time during her long night shifts but she also offered to do some cleaning and laundry while Brad slept. Emali prepared meals for Brad—who was eating a limited diet at that time in addition to his nightly intravenous nutrition—and eventually for our family, including a fantastic Fijian chicken curry that we all loved.

Over the course of that summer I paid Nancy and Emali a total of about $40,000, not a penny of it covered by insurance. I worried constantly I wasn't paying them enough for their service. Being able to afford their help means I'm probably in the top 1 percent of privilege for caregivers, for which I'm deeply thankful. I was and am also frustrated that such care isn't covered by insurance. It's a bitter irony, since in-home healthcare is enormously cheaper than hospitalization—and good home assistance can prevent the falls, injuries, or infections that could easily land a fragile patient right back in the hospital.

Brad's health insurance, which is wildly generous by US standards, provided for a skilled nursing visit twice weekly (mainly to take a blood draw for labs) and a short visit from a "home health nurse" three times a week. The home health service was frustrating to use in practice, however—the workers were meant to help with showering, dressing, and toileting, and not much else. The times when they could come were unpredictable and very hard to schedule in the midst of all of Brad's other services. Sometimes they showed up at the wrong times or not at all. In the end I told the home health agency not to come anymore. The workers we were paying directly were easier to manage and vastly more helpful.

Every time I think about the relative costs of different types of healthcare, it blows my mind. I once received an Explanation of Benefits statement showing that the billed services for a few weeks in the BMTU were more than $3 million.[7] It seems shocking that the medical system can't spare dollar figures in the thousands to pay for professional in-home care. If a medical professional tells the family that the patient has a medical need for twenty-four-hour attendance, as Dr. T did, it doesn't make sense that that very attendance is a noncovered expense.[8] For that matter, why can't insurance or the state pay family caregivers providing medically necessary care?

I'd estimate that my caregiving in the summer of 2016 took up at least thirty hours a week and likely more. For the first several weeks after Brad's discharge I was on eight to ten phone calls a day related to his care. My time went to tasks that care workers couldn't do: calling insurance, sorting out bills, applying for Social Security disability insurance, working with HR to untangle bureaucratic knots, scheduling appointments, calling the transplant advice nurse with concerns. Brad's vision loss was a complicating factor. He couldn't reliably use his phone and struggled with adaptive technology. Communicating with him if I had to be out of the house was difficult. I also found that, compared to the person I'd known before his illness, Brad seemed cognitively impaired: not as sharp, not as able to track details. That was an understandable impairment given the number of his medications and the megadoses of chemo he'd endured, but it was a frustrating one.

Speaking of those medications, just keeping track of them was a challenge. Many were specialty items that had to go through the Cancer Center pharmacy at his medical group, which didn't offer automatic refills, and none of them ran out at the same time so I had to check almost daily on what he might need soon. Some of them had to be picked up at specific, scheduled times. A few of his prescriptions were so rare that they demanded high-level special handling and could come only through a mail-order compounding pharmacy (a thing I hadn't known existed).

Brad's TPN kits came in enormous, heavy boxes delivered weekly by courier, with bags of fluid and liquid vitamin mix that had to be injected into the bags just before hooking up the pump every night. The pump ran for ten hours nightly, providing about half of Brad's caloric needs as he slept. The kits included everything for the hookup—including a fresh 9-volt battery for each night and a quarter to open the battery case—and had to be unpacked and refrigerated as soon as they arrived. Every time I unpacked one or fussed with that tricky pump, I seethed about that senior physician's comment that "you just plug it in."

The amount of medical waste we generated was astounding. I tried to dispose of medications and sharps responsibly but it's hard to find drops for those; many places that said they accepted used sharps or medications on, say, their website were baffled when I turned up, and refused to take them. I was becoming less and less patient with small, frustrating incidents like that—a telling sign of burnout. With every small obstacle, every fresh demand, every fifteen-minute delay at the oncologist's office, every extra person in my house, I felt a rising wave of hot irritation that I was struggling more and more to contain.

BONE BROTH

One June morning a few weeks after Brad came home, I was pouring myself a too-big iced coffee when his physical therapist beckoned me urgently into our dining room. It was 9 a.m. and I had been up for four hours, in which time I had fed the kids breakfast, made lunches, answered some emails, unhooked Brad from his pump, showered, eaten breakfast standing up in the kitchen, walked the kids to school, spoken to the principal about the six-year-old's class assignment for next year, and returned home, sweaty and already tired. The day's predicted high temperature was 106 degrees. Besides Brad and me, the people in the house included Emali, the physical therapist, the social worker, and the occupational therapist.

Even on a good day, the physical therapist drove me bananas. Her husband had also undergone a stem cell transplant. She was thus sure she knew more than I about everything I was going through as a caregiver—though her husband's case had been different, uncomplicated by GvHD—and was always sharing tips. The urgency of her calling me in, though, made me think there was an emergency.

"Oh, there you are," she said—implying, to my raw feelings, that I'd been insufficiently responsive. "I'm writing down the instructions for making bone broth. It would be really good for his gut health and you should be making it for him."

"Excuse me?" I said.

"Bone broth," she repeated, gesturing at the page. "Or your caregiver could make it."

"I do make him broth," I said, gripping my glass so tightly my hand shook.

"But do you make *bone* broth? It's long-extracted and it has special properties," she said. "It restored my husband's nutritional status when he had his transplant."

All broth is fucking bone broth, I did not say out loud. Calling it bone broth is a fad, I did not say out loud. I had started making Brad broth when he was in the hospital. I went to a special butcher shop to get stewing hens to make it stronger and more protein-rich. In fact, I'd placed a short little article in a local magazine that month about where to find the best chicken to make the best broth—just about the only thing I'd published that year. It felt like the physical therapist was not only questioning my domestic skills but erasing my entire professional identity. Her well-intentioned question unleashed something in me much as the bat had done.

What I did say out loud was this: "You know, people tell me I need to be doing something for other people all day long, every day." I didn't mask my irritation and I hoped she'd take the hint.

"It's a *suggestion*," she said in faux-calm, soothing tones, as if I were a feral cat trapped in a small space, which is how I felt. "For when you have time. I think you'll find it very helpful."

My rage boiled over like unattended broth. "I have to go," I said, stalking into my kitchen, where Emali and the social worker from the rehab company were standing. In the living room sat Brad and the occupational therapist. I felt boxed in, especially because my desk was in the kitchen. The physical therapist followed me.

"I was only trying to help," she said.

"Why don't you stick to, you know, doing physical therapy?" I said, knowing I was being rude, and the rehab team would discuss me later as That Wife, but I was too mad to shut up. "My husband is being followed by three dietitians. They can tell me if I really need to make him broth."

"Good nutrition is an essential part of physical recovery," she continued blandly.

That did it. "You know what? If anybody in this whole situation gave enough of a shit about me to even ask what it is I do, you might know that in my professional life I'm a food writer and recipe developer and I actually know something about broth. But I'm not really a person anymore, I guess."

"Well!" Now she was offended. "I was *only* trying to help." But I was already on my way out the back door, which I slammed hard enough that its elderly panes of glass rattled. I stomped down the block. When I returned, sweaty, the social worker was still there. I spent the rest of the morning venting to him and sobbing on the back porch. It was tremendously cathartic but I remained a ball of tense anger for most of that summer.

Up until then I'd kept most of my caregiver anger sternly repressed or talked about it only in my therapist's office. What chafed the most was not the private demands from my husband, but the public, official ones from nurses, doctors, and therapists, many of whom seemed to discount my personhood in any other realm than as a caregiver. I wanted them to recognize my humanity. I felt, on every level, unseen in my life, even as I was holding together the lives of four people. The longer I acted as a caregiver, the angrier I found myself at that erasure.

My anger started to flare often at home, where I could hardly rein in my irritation, even at the smallest details. The plump wet pink sponge on the side of the sink, for instance, made me grit my teeth every day. Whenever I squeezed it, it disgorged dishwatery fluid, teeming with bacteria. When Brad used the sponge, he was too weak to wring it out all the way. The sponge festered unless I noticed it was too pink, too moist, and gave it another squeeze with my stronger grip, draining it as completely as Brad's long illness drained me. My frustration with an unsqueezed sponge was not just housewifely pettiness. Everything at our house needed to be sanitary; Brad's doctors had him on three different types of immune suppressants to combat the complications of his transplant. Frequently, I sniffed the sponge to find a telltale whiff of mildew and threw it in the trash a little harder than necessary.

When I got out each new sponge I always carefully closed the doors under the sink. One has a protruding lip, so you have to close them in order or else the left one stands ajar. This is a minor detail of my house that the other people who were in and out during Brad's illness—home healthcare workers, relatives there to help out—consistently failed to notice when they took out a trash bag or refilled the hand-soap dispenser. They were helping me, doing tasks that otherwise would have been mine. Every time I found the door ajar, it represented one less bag of trash I had to carry outside and replace with a fresh bag, one less sponge I had to get out when the old one had gone smelly. Yet when I saw the door ajar I was seized by illogical resentment.

The minor details of domestic life seem petty to me even as I enumerate them. But my extreme irritation at the stupid sponge and cabinet doors masked a deeper sense of loss about our daily lives. The sponge reminded me of how meticulous Brad had once been about the dishes. If I left the sponge wet he would hold it up and declaim a line from *Hamlet*: "Take you me for a sponge?" I missed the husband who could make private jokes from Shakespeare when we argued about doing the dishes. The texture of our lives had come from such small priorities, daily choices, and habits.

When Brad got sick all this was rinsed away. But I couldn't afford the time to mourn. Part of me worried that if I stopped to really process those feelings of loss I would fall into an irrecoverable grief. I didn't have time: I had groceries to buy, children to raise, a husband's life to save. Anger was easier than my real feelings: terror of widowhood and abandonment. Sadness that cancer had fractured our lives just when it seemed like things were getting good—we had become financially stable, the kids had grown old enough to give us time to ourselves, and Brad's professional duties had eased. Every time I thought about the family life that we'd lost, I wanted to cry. But if I started to cry, it seemed like I might never stop, so I stuffed those feelings down, crossed more items off my always-growing to-do list, and powered through. Anger kept me moving, even as its heat was contributing to my growing burnout. Sometimes it pushed me right out the door. Sometimes I found ways to go numb.

LIPSTICK ON A SHOT GLASS

Brad was trying to reenter our family as the partner and parent he had once been, but in truth he was not physically up to the task. The first thing he tried doing was a few dishes. His visual impairment and physical weakness meant he couldn't see things he spilled or smears on dishes, such as the lipstick smudge on the Hillary Clinton campaign shot glass I picked up one night to fill with bourbon. "Made from 100% shattered glass ceiling," it read.

For a time, eating and drinking were among the only things I did for pleasure, but even those were often out of my control. Dozens of generous friends and acquaintances and even a few strangers brought us meals, which I ate gratefully while hardly even noticing what they were. I bought wine based on the preferences of my in-laws when they were staying with us, not my own. But I bought bourbon for myself and switched to that at night after my in-laws had gone to bed. Most of the liquor was downstairs on the bar in the basement, built by former owners who had hosted legendary parties, but the bourbon I kept on the main floor so that I could grab a shot or two after whoever was staying in the basement—my in-laws during Brad's hospitalization, Brad after he came home—had gone to bed.

Most nights I poured myself some bourbon in one shot glass or another. That is, when I didn't swig it directly from the bottle. My overall drinking crept up during the years of Brad's illness. "I'm still at less than a bottle a day," I said to a friend. I was referring to wine, I should point out, and she thought that sounded pretty reasonable under the circumstances.

"I'll enable you now," she said, "and I'll help you quit when you need to when all this is over. It's very effective for anxiety."

As Brad got sicker and sicker, I began drinking a bit more, and a bit more, each night. I worried about it. I come from a family of heavy drinkers; three of my grandparents could probably have been called functional alcoholics. None of them ever wrecked their life or hit rock bottom but I wondered whether I wanted to spend my life as deeply in thrall to alcohol as they had.

I began to bargain with myself. It wasn't so bad, I reasoned, if I wasn't drinking during the day. A glass of wine at lunch wasn't so bad, once a week or so. A couple, no three, no four, in the evening wasn't so bad. If I never let myself go. If I never acted weird. If the kids couldn't tell. If I stayed reliable. If I never put booze in my morning coffee or drank before noon. (I didn't.) If I didn't drink from the bottle. (I let that one go.) If I stayed below some arbitrary amount every day. If I could quit when Brad got better. If he got better.

Ah, fuck it, I said to myself too often as I poured another shot or took a swig. I started to think of myself as the phlegmatic, stoic Grace Poole, the bad caregiver of *Jane Eyre*. Jane mentions Grace often has a "pot of porter" to make her job tolerable. Who wouldn't, hired to keep a madwoman quiet in an uncomfortable attic? I drank to keep my rage under control, to quiet myself. I was Bertha and Grace and Jane (in crude Freudian terms, id and ego and superego) all in one.

In public and during the day I tried to present as a good caregiver, but over the course of Brad's illness, and especially after he came home from the transplant, my house became less and less a private refuge and more and more a public, medical space. At the same time, my burnout was growing. I felt frantic, as surveilled as Bertha Mason yet as overlooked as Jane Eyre.

I felt—from nurses, from acquaintances, from relatives, from Brad, from myself, from nearly everyone except my therapist and a few beloved friends—constant pressure to be sunny and upbeat. I came to detest the clichés offered by the well-meaning: stay positive. You got this. I couldn't be as strong as you are. You have to stay strong for him. What doesn't kill you makes you stronger. Hang in there (complete with the mental image of a scrabbling kitten on a 1980s poster). God doesn't give you more than you can handle. Everything happens for a reason. (For anyone who's ever felt put off by such admonitions, there's now a significant cultural backlash, as seen with Emily McDowell's series of realistic "empathy cards" or the withering critique of positivity culture in Barbara Ehrenreich's *Bright-Sided*.[9])

In response, I wanted to scream or turn sullen: I don't, actually, have to stay positive, I wanted to answer. Even if my time was no longer my own, surely my feelings could be. I felt like I was constantly performing a version of Good Caregiver, Good Mom, or Good Woman. I wished I'd had the presence of mind—or willingness to be rude—of Kate Bowler's husband in her cancer memoir *Everything Happens for a Reason (And Other Lies I've Loved)*: "A neighbor knocked on our door to tell my husband that everything happens for a reason. 'I'd love to hear it,' my husband said. 'Pardon?' she said, startled. 'I'd love to hear the reason my wife is dying,' he said, in that sweet and sour way he has, effectively ending the conversation as the neighbor stammered something and handed him a casserole."[10]

Sweet and sour: that's a feeling I identify with. I always aimed for a polite tone with hidden acerbity in response to the well-meaning people. Bowler's book, naturally, focuses on the perspective of a patient, not a caregiver, but is a thoughtful exploration of some of the cultural ideas around tragedies and illness—cancer in particular, but any, really—that plagued me as a caregiver. She outlines the "minimizers," people who say "at least" (at least you have resources, at least it's not worse); the "teachers" who want her to find a lesson in her travails; and the "Solutions People," like one woman who writes to her, "'Keep smiling! Your attitude determines your destiny.'" Bowler is "worn out by the tyranny of prescriptive joy," a phenomenon I, too, hated.[11] Even my own father (usually a reliably sardonic presence) told me offhandedly that I "had to stay positive."

I felt furious and kept it barely suppressed, all the time. Is this, I wondered, what it was like to be a Victorian woman? I felt like I was wearing an emotional corset. At night was the only time I could loosen the corset. I put my hair up, wiped off my lipstick, took off my bra, grabbed a handful of cookies or chocolate, and poured bourbon in a shot glass. I took my nightcap up to my room like Grace Poole, whose job is mainly to keep Bertha Mason quiet, though she fails: Jane often hears creepy laughter, and a crisis of the book comes when Bertha escapes the attic and rips the veil Jane was to have worn for her wedding.

INVISIBLE LABOR

At first the social worker on the rehab team had been unsure of how he could best help us. His job was to assess family and social factors that contribute to or inhibit the patient's recovery, and see how he could support the patient given those factors. Brad, with a strong network of family support and economic stability, seemed less in need of that. (There was already a psychotherapist on the team dedicated to providing talk therapy for him.) But after the social worker saw me melt down in response to the physical therapist and realized how distant Brad and I were from each other, he offered us marriage counseling. Honestly, it was a challenge. I didn't really want to be there, doing more work to keep my relationship with Brad—such as it was then—alive. I felt like I had to beg to have my labor recognized, and for what? Unless I left my husband it wasn't as if I could stop being his caregiver, or hand over responsibility for the kids to him, or say, "Here, you cook dinner for once." Even the idea of leaving him felt like too much work.

My emotional needs at the time were in direct contradiction to each other: I was torn between wanting to be left severely alone and wanting to be seen and supported—loved, really—in an entirely different way than my life permitted. These two desires were a paradox that I still don't know how to reconcile. That poor social worker; he did his best, and I think he helped, but our relationship crisis was, I think, beyond almost anyone's powers to fix at that time. (We've gone on to defeat at least one other couples counselor since; the jury's still out on the one we're seeing as of this writing.)

As part of his efforts to rebuild our relationship, the social worker once asked what we loved about each other. Brad replied: "I've always loved and appreciated the life Kate has made for me." He was referring to our home, in which I chose nearly every object; to our children, whom he was initially less sure he wanted; to trips we've taken, how we celebrate holidays, the brand of sugar we buy.

I understood what he meant but that well-intentioned answer pissed me off in ways he hadn't expected. In my angry state it came across not as appreciation but as an assumption that my goal in life had been to support Brad and make his life better.

"That's just it," I snapped back. "I didn't do it for you. I made the life I wanted for me. You've been along for the ride." Like many other things I said then, this was unfair, but contained kernels of truth: I had made our lives for me but also for us and our children. But he seemed to accept many of the conditions of our life together as simple tribute. What must it be like, I wondered, to show up on a vacation simply trusting that there would be airline tickets, a rental car, a hotel room, all planned and ready for you to step into? To know that whatever breaks in the house will be fixed? To know dinner will appear and the mortgage will be paid? How carefree, but how alienating. Talk about something not being your beautiful life.

Is there any such thing as an equitable marriage? I'm sure there is but it's hard to come by. There's been a spate of books recently and popular debates asking this question, especially around issues of parenthood. Like my generational peers—many of whom are currently turning out books with titles like *Fed Up*, *Women's Work*, and *All the Rage*—I discovered over years of marriage that parenthood, especially, tilted the balance of labor toward me.

Caregiving tipped the nonbalance even further. Having little to no identity outside of caregiving frustrated me even more than a similar dynamic had when I became a mother. Even motherhood hadn't been so consuming, hadn't erased me so thoroughly. To this day friends and acquaintances tend to ask me how Brad is before they ask how I am. So I've appreciated the recent flowering of books about motherhood, work/life balance, and the challenges faced by women. We need a similar clamor of voices about eldercare and caregiving for the ill—the often forgotten, even less glamorous analogues of childcare. Although male participation in caregiving is growing, women still most often bear the brunt of it. The coronavirus pandemic of 2020, when suddenly kids were home all the time, highlighted and even exacerbated those inequities, as British journalist Helen Lewis wrote in a piece for *The Atlantic* baldly titled "The Coronavirus Is a Disaster for Feminism": "What do pandemic patients need? Looking after. What do self-isolating older people need? Looking after. What do children kept home from school need? Looking after. All this looking after—this unpaid caring labor—will fall more heavily on women, because of the existing structure of the workforce."[12]

Like my mother before me I became a contract worker—a freelancer, though I chose that path somewhat more freely than she did. But I, too, followed my husband's job and fortunes. My work was fungible and flexible and, in the end, dispensable. I was the one making plans for the kids, shopping for and swapping out their clothes, taking the day off when one was sick, decluttering, paying all the bills and doing all the paperwork, furnishing and maintaining the house, cooking dinner, making travel plans, planning all our socializing. Brad had long had a few default tasks (taking out the garbage, giving the flea drops to the cat), and before his cancer was usually open to delegated tasks, but underneath it all he assumed that nearly everything was my job unless otherwise negotiated. Indeed, so many of the things I did were tasks he didn't even realize were happening, like sorting and cleaning out the kids' clothes, season after season, year after year. Other things seemed equal enough to him because he conveniently didn't notice how much labor was attached to what I did. For instance, he did his own laundry. I also, of course, did my own laundry. But when the kids were little, who did he think was washing all of their clothes, the sheets, the towels? To be honest, I think he thought changing sheets was just an odd compulsion I had, if he ever thought about it at all.

Over the years before his illness, cooking had become a particular bone of contention. I was twenty-three when we moved in together and we agreed that I would cook and he would clean up. I liked cooking and was good at it; he hated it and found it intimidating, so it seemed like an equal trade. And cooking, in the guise of recipe development, had become part of my work when I transitioned to a career as a food writer after graduate school, so there was a logic in me being the cook. But the workload around planning and executing seven dinners a week (even with occasional takeout) grew with our family. That mental load made the tasks completely disproportionate, as essayist and columnist Zoe Fenson points out in her incisive piece "It's So Much More Than Cooking" in *The Week*.[13]

One night at the dinner table, months before Brad was seriously ill, I was declaiming to him and the girls about everything I did, everything they should appreciate, everything I keep track of. I was up on a high horse. They said, "What are you talking about? What do you mean, you're keeping track of everything?" I answered them by talking for five minutes, and I ended by saying I was keeping track of the chairs. They laughed at me. Keeping track of the chairs? In the dining room? The chairs are always there. What is there to track? I said, these chairs aren't great and we only have four in the matched set, so I'm always half-looking for better ones that match the table so I can swap them in, and monitoring when it's time to replace the little pads on the bottom of the legs. They laughed again, and it's true—maybe keeping track of immobile chairs isn't the most demanding job. But multiply that out across every piece of furniture, every food item in the fridge, the oil levels in the car, the fourteen (I counted) kinds of light bulbs that various fixtures in our home demand, whether the kids have enough socks—the job becomes enormous.

The problem, as Megan K. Stack notes in her book *Women's Work*, is every single one of these responsibilities is too goddamn petty to make a fuss about. "No single task is ever worth the argument," Stack writes. "Scrub a toilet, wash a few dishes, respond to the note from the teacher, talk to another mother, buy the supplies. Don't make a big deal out of everything. Don't make a big deal out of anything. Never mind that, writ large, all these minor chores are the reason we remain stuck in this depressing hole of pointless conversations and stifled accomplishment."[14] The smallness of each single task bakes in a partner's ironclad defense: you're making a big deal about nothing. You're so silly, little lady, with your wish to keep track of those immobile chairs and act like that's a real thing. But such an attitude ignores the fact that everyone has to sit on something to eat the dinner I made.

. . .

If one person amid that "everyone" in the family falls seriously ill, I quickly found, those petty demands shoot up with alarming quickness. Someone—more often than not a woman—must take on the mental labor of planning and the emotional strain of caring. Society assumes she will do it gladly and then dismisses her from its mind. A generation before me, women might have been quietly annoyed by the demands of such caring but they had been raised to think the domestic was naturally their sphere. I grew up wanting and expecting more and was unwilling to remain invisible. Through no fault of Brad's, when he came home from the hospital we were in a zero-sum game in which his needs and wants inevitably subtracted from mine. I resisted thinking of him as a burden rather than a valued, beloved person—an ableist trap that is all too common in the discourse of caregiving—but I regret to say that for some time the weight of caring was almost all I could see in our relationship. I carried that weight almost invisibly, as is the way of caregivers. By the middle of that summer, though, I was so fried and frazzled that what I wanted more than anything else was to disappear myself—to flee. It was a sign of just how burned out I'd become.

FIVE

TO A CRISP

Burnout

I knew I was burned out well before I took that quiz that told me I was already toast, but seeing it on the computer screen drove the point home. During that summer after Brad came home from the hospital the signs were unmistakable: I was irritable all the time, ready to snap at the slightest provocation. I was impatient with my slow-moving, ill husband and I wasn't nice to him about it, either. I felt hemmed in on every side, thwarted at every turn, and although I kept the household running and all the metaphorical balls in the air, I don't think anyone enjoyed my company, least of all me.

Even though I was angry when my husband's doctor told me, "If you don't take care of yourself, you can't take care of him," there was a lot of truth in it, as there is in the saying about putting on your own oxygen mask first. What I couldn't articulate to him, or even to myself in the middle of my rage-crying storm, was that I needed help and care and real relief regardless of whether it made me a better caregiver; I needed it because I was a person.

Burnout kills empathy and makes worse caregivers of all of us who suffer from it. More than that, it made me a worse person: less kind, less patient, less fun to be around. Being so depleted made me miserable and being miserable made me, frankly, a bitch. The trouble is that if you're burned out you can't take care of yourself very effectively, either. I was coping as best I could: going to the gym, trying to get enough sleep, maintaining a few supportive friendships—at least by text and online. But during the summer of 2016, often the only solution I found for my burnout was to leave home at every opportunity.

FLEEING

It wasn't easy to get away from home, despite all the help I had marshalled for Brad. There were our daughters to consider as well. (I discuss the challenges of so-called sandwiched caregiving in more depth in chapter 7.) The end of the school year is always a time with lots of demands on parents: open houses, performances, early dismissals, fundraising events, last-minute projects. I remember having to hastily borrow a little red wagon from neighbors and then panic-order a plastic lobster on Amazon for Nora's mini float representing Massachusetts in the fifth-grade parade of the states.

By the time school got out in mid-June, I had more than hit my limit. I was really, really looking forward to the week of sleepaway camp I'd signed the girls up for—Camp Kesem. One of the girls' therapists had told me about the camp, which is specifically for kids ages six to seventeen who are affected by a parent's cancer. Our daughter Lucy, then six, turned out to be the youngest girl in her session of the camp by two years, and I was a little nervous about sending her so young, but I couldn't wait for the break. Five whole nights without the girls sounded like bliss. Brad wanted us to spend more time together, but I wanted to get the hell away from everyone. Nancy and Emali had been with us for more than a month by then and were able to handle all of Brad's routines, and they were fine with me leaving for a bit. I booked a couple of nights at a spalike resort in Calistoga, all by myself, to unwind. It was as good as it sounded. I read, swam, and rested, and then I returned home with dread.

As soon as I set foot back in the house I was swamped again with the feeling of being overwhelmed. Everywhere were reminders of how completely illness dominated our lives, from the medications cluttering our dining room to the white cane leaning by the door. Brad was starting slowly to recover a bit of independence and thanks to the cane he could go out for walks (which always worried me even as I was glad to see him pushing himself in his recovery). His social calendar was starting to be busier than mine; his old friends and colleagues rallied to visit him, adding more people to our already overcrowded house. One poet friend of his came to our house faithfully, always bringing poetry to read aloud sonorously, wearing jangly jewelry and a hefty dose of musky perfume; I started making excuses to flee the scene when she was there. More and more, however, Brad was getting adept at taking walks and he occasionally met friends at nearby coffee shops. He returned home from his excursions exhausted but satisfied, and I was the opposite: I returned home from my short trips well rested but unhappy to be back.

Sometimes leaving home backfired on me, as it did over Fourth of July weekend. Our holiday tradition had been to go to our shared family cabin in the mountains above my hometown. Old family friends with their own cabin nearby hosted an annual party that we usually went to; the year before, I had taken the girls but Brad had stayed home, recovering from chemo. In 2016, he was even less able to travel, but I took the girls for what I hoped would be a respite in the mountains. I hadn't reckoned on how overwhelming it would be to join a big family gathering. The cabin was more packed than usual that year; several members of my sister-in-law's large family came for the first time and friends of my brother's drove up for the day. The small cabin was stretched past its capacity, without enough beds for everyone, and the kids kept each other awake late into the night. I felt brittle and ambushed. Everyone asked about Brad, so I had to repeat the complex, ambiguous story of how he was doing over and over while friends said it was great he was doing so well. Nobody ever seemed to grasp just how fragile he was, nor how tenuously I was coping. That getaway ended up feeling far more stressful than staying at home would have been.

The biggest trip of that summer—the hardest won and most intricately planned—was, like the cabin visit, partly for the girls' sake and partly for my own. That was the year *Hamilton* hit it big. The preceding October, before I had any inkling of how the stem cell transplant would go, three friends and I had bought the earliest available tickets to the Broadway show—which proved to be in August, ten months later. The four of us made a plan to meet in New York for the show no matter what. I'm not normally a Broadway fan but something about the intense fad for *Hamilton* that year swept me up in it, perhaps in part as escapism: I followed Lin-Manuel Miranda on Twitter, watched the stage-door videos the cast made, hoped I could keep the promise to meet my friends to see it, hoped we'd get to see the original cast. In the spring I set about trying to figure out how to make it happen.

I knew that the girls badly wanted to visit Brad's parents in western Quebec that summer—my in-laws have a cottage on a small lake there and the girls loved their yearly kayaking, hiking in the woods, and swimming with Nana and Grampa. We had missed going the year before when Brad was in chemo. With my in-laws' considerable help we wrapped both the New York and Canada trips into one eastward swing. Joe took over my caregiving duties with Brad in California while the girls and I flew first to Ottawa (the closest airport to the lake) and stayed a few days with Susan. I then flew to New York by myself, met up with my friends and saw the show, and then flew to Toronto, where I met Susan and the girls, and we visited Brad's brother and his family.

It was an ambitious, tiring trip, and looking back I can't quite fathom how I had the wherewithal to put it together, but that time with friends—just for fun and just for me—gave an immense lift to my mental state in that intense summer. The trip also gave me something crucial during the stressful spring months in which Brad transitioned from hospital and to home: something to look forward to. Recovering from a state of burnout isn't easy, and even now, years later, I find myself still affected by that period of extreme depletion of my care resources. (I write more about those longer-term effects of caregiving in chapters 8 and 9.) But my instincts to flee the situation, which I often felt bad about in those days, were self-preserving.

WHY WE'RE BURNED OUT

As a burned-out caregiver I was far from alone, and many of my fellow burnouts have little chance of finding much respite. Why is family caregiving such a strain for so many in the US? Answering that demands a closer look at who caregivers are and what they—or rather we—are actually doing. Gender and race are major factors in the relative stress caregivers experience. As we've seen, the majority of family caregivers in the US are women: our ranks by most analyses are as much as 75 percent female.[1] Female caregivers typically spend more time caring for their charges than males do, about twenty-two hours per week on average versus seventeen.

(In some good news for millennial women, however, the gender gap appears to be closing among younger caregivers.)[2] There are also significant disparities in the intensity of the caregiving tasks that male and female caregivers take on. Studies show that female caregivers take on the most difficult tasks—such as toileting assistance—more frequently than men, who "are more likely to help with finances, arrangement of care, and other less burdensome tasks."[3] Women may also be more likely to stick around for intense or long-term caregiving: a 2009 study in the journal *Cancer* found that fewer than 3 percent of women left a male spouse suffering such a serious illness, while 21 percent of male caregivers abandoned their female partners.[4]

The average age of caregivers in the United States is forty-nine. Perhaps not coincidentally, this figure is not far from the age—47.2 years—given as the developed world's "peak of unhappiness" in a recent study by Dartmouth economist David Blanchflower. The study tracked the so-called U-curve of happiness across a lifetime, a theory I first encountered in Ada Calhoun's *Why We Can't Sleep*.[5] Although Blanchflower doesn't delve into the reasons for this dip, he comments that it corresponds with his personal experience (he was in his late sixties at the time of the study), and as several analysts have commented, caregiving likely plays a role: people in their late forties are most likely to be caught between caring for elderly parents and young children.[6] Calhoun further points out that Generation X is particularly squeezed when it comes to caregiving: we are part of a "baby bust" and thus are likely to have fewer siblings to pitch in with eldercare; our parents are more likely than those of other generations to have divorced, meaning we may have multiple parental households to care for; and we've delayed having children, meaning we have younger kids at home as our parents enter old age (a factor I'll look at in more depth in chapter 7).[7]

Of course, it's not all on Generation X: plenty of millennials and boomers are caregivers as well, with the number of millennials in those roles growing fast. A composite image of a "typical" millennial caregiver, published by the National Alliance for Caregiving and AARP, presents a twenty-seven-year-old who spends twenty-one hours a week caring for an older female relative—either a parent or a grandparent.[8] (That's in addition to having a full-time job.) Just under half of caregivers are between eighteen and forty-nine years of age and just over a third are older than sixty-five. Interestingly—and sadly—the number of hours dedicated to caregiving increases among older caregivers, presumably indicating higher needs among older recipients. Older caregivers are more likely to be caring for a partner and to be experiencing declining health themselves. Caring for an elderly parent represents a plurality of caregiving situations (42 percent), and the average age of care recipients (65 percent of whom are female) is sixty-nine.

The gender balance of caregivers is reversed in the LGBTQ community, which makes up about 9 percent of caregivers. (Note: this statistic is not broken out for transgender caregivers.) In this group, gay male caregivers report spending more hours on care than their lesbian counterparts and vastly more hours on care (forty-one) than straight male caregivers (twenty-nine). In all, 14 percent of gay men report they are full-time caregivers. The care needs of the elderly LGBTQ community may be particularly acute, as members of this population are twice as likely to live alone as their straight counterparts and three to four times less likely to have children. According to the National LGBT Cancer Network, "LGBT caregivers are far more likely to be friends and 'chosen family' to the person they care for, rather than partners or biological family members."[9] Many observers and studies point to the horrific losses of the HIV/AIDS crisis—especially the paranoia surrounding AIDS among straight communities—as a key factor in the development of strong communal care networks.[10] Medical discrimination against the LGBTQ community, unfortunately, continues: a 2011 study shows that up to 20 percent of older LGBT individuals and a staggering 44 percent of transgender individuals fear they won't receive equitable medical care if their health provider knows their sexual orientation or gender identity—suggesting a special need for sensitivity and advocacy from caregivers.[11]

The National LGBT Cancer Network's website identifies the HIV/AIDS crisis as "the origin of a culture of mutual caregiving within the LGBT community." This shift was a matter of necessity: "Blatant discrimination against LGBT individuals, and fears and stigma about HIV/AIDS among the general population and healthcare workers thrust caregiving upon LGBT friends of the ill as a cultural imperative that continues today."[12] Rebecca Makkai's 2018 novel *The Great Believers* (which I also discuss in chapter 8) depicts the development of just such a community network of chosen family.[13] Similar care networks can come together when communities mobilize and "break out the spreadsheets" to offer collective support to trans individuals undergoing gender-confirming surgery—critical for people who may be estranged from their families of origin.[14] Such networks could be an inspiring model for easing burnout among overstretched primary caregivers in all communities as the care gap becomes more acute.

The racial and ethnic breakdown of caregivers is 62 percent white, 13 percent African American, 17 percent Latinx,[15] and 6 percent Asian American—not far off from the percentages of each group in the population as a whole.[16] What is more telling than those raw statistics, however, is the prevalence of caregiving within each of those categories. White Americans had the lowest prevalence of caregivers, with 16.9 percent of whites acting as caregivers in 2015. The Latinx and Black populations have the highest prevalence of caregivers: 21 percent and 20.3 percent, respectively. African American and Latinx caregivers were on average also younger—forty-four and forty-two years old, respectively—than their white (52.5) and Asian American (46.6) counterparts. Those numbers suggest that cultural and economic pressures, as well as lower overall life expectancies and a greater prevalence of health problems, push people in these groups into unpaid caregiving roles earlier and at higher rates. The number of Black family caregivers is expected to triple by 2030.[17] The Family Caregiver Alliance also estimates Black and Latinx caregivers "experience higher burdens from caregiving and spend more time caregiving on average than their white or Asian American peers."[18] Glenn likewise notes nonwhite women are more likely to be sandwiched by caregiving responsibilities: "Women of color, especially African American women, are more likely to have to combine elder and disabled care with employment outside the home," a profound stressor.[19]

The distinct challenges facing nonwhite caregivers resonate painfully with the traumatic legacy of American slavery, in which Black women were forced to care for white slaveholders and their families while being separated from their own. After slavery, as Anne-Marie Slaughter points out in *Unfinished Business*, Black American women were often locked into underpaid care work: "For generations of African American women, caregiving and breadwinning have been the same thing; they have earned their living and supported or helped support their own families by caring for other people's families."[20] Other women of color and immigrant women have also long been shunted into low-paid or unpaid exploitive caring labor, a shameful history ripe for redress. As Slaughter notes, "Starting from the perspective of care would place a much higher value on the work that women of color have traditionally done."[21]

Just as many kinds of emotional, mental, social, and domestic tasks make up the invisible labor of the working woman's famed "second shift," so do countless types of work constitute caregiving. Any overview of care labor will leave out some tasks, and no individual experience can represent all. Broadly, though, caregiving can be broken down into categories of tasks and responsibilities, some more taxing than others.

Across the spectrum of eldercare, childcare, care for the ill, and other domestic caring labor, Glenn identifies three main types of activities, which she notes are inseparable.[22] All come into play in caregiving for the ill, but the first, "direct caring," predominates. This category includes physical tending; emotional care, such as "offering reassurance"; and services to meet basic needs, such as grocery shopping. Most common is direct care involving help with "activities of daily living" (ADLs), such as dressing, bathing, grooming, and getting in and out of bed. Nearly all family caregivers perform these tasks, though, as noted above, there are gender disparities in this category, with women tending to take on more grueling jobs.

Personal assistance with such private tasks as toileting is an especially demanding form of direct care, which can provoke shame and mixed feelings for both caregiver and recipient—a worry that Brad and I had, as I've noted, after his transplant. But it's not just spouses who can struggle with this kind of labor: the role reversal of parent-child dynamics in eldercare can be particularly painful, especially if the relationship is already strained. We get a visceral look at how upsetting such caregiving can be in Gwendolyn Brooks's poem "Jessie Mitchell's Mother," in which the two title characters are deeply at odds. The daughter goes "Into her mother's bedroom to wash the ballooning body," thinking dismissively of her mother's "brain of jelly" and reflecting that she won't cry if the mother dies. Old divides, based on the mother's colorism (the mother takes pride in being lighter skinned than her daughter), further strain the caregiving relationship.[23] Brooks's poem also suggests another element of stress in caregiving: the old patterns, hurts, and challenges of a relationship do not vanish when one party needs care. As I often found, on a stressful day with Brad it was hard to ignore old frustrations and easy to remember times

I felt he had failed to care for me. I tried not to let such memories fester into resentment but they inevitably added to emotional strain.

Perhaps a less fraught form of caregiving is one Glenn calls her second category: "maintaining the immediate physical surroundings" in which care recipients live, such as doing laundry or sweeping the floor. Some ADL assistance fits into this category, and 72 percent of caregivers assist with housework.[24] Maintaining physical surroundings can be fraught too. In *Demystifying Hospice*, for instance, author Karen J. Clayton tells the story of a caregiver she visits, Gerry, who is overwhelmed by the delivery of needed medical furniture.[25] She is agitated because she needs to rearrange the house to accommodate things for her husband's care, a situation I remember well. When Brad was about to come home from the hospital, an acquaintance from my gym, an occasional lifting partner, asked what she could do to help. I asked her to come over and move furniture with me to get the house ready for Brad's return.

A third category Glenn names, kin work, is "the work of fostering people's relationships and social connections."[26] That may not seem much like labor, but arranging visits, communicating with distant family about medical decisions, replying to texts from friends about how everyone is doing: all of these things take time. Care recipients vary widely in their ability to keep up these connections for themselves, as Brad's case showed me plainly. At times, as when he was undergoing inpatient chemo but feeling relatively well, he was terribly bored and wanted to arrange visits with family and friends. Later, when he was at his sickest, he was unable to receive visitors, but that was when people were most likely to inquire after him. I couldn't blame them but I had no mental space to update dozens of people. When he lost his vision he was no longer able to use his phone with ease and his connection to the outside world eroded still further. I was glad I had convinced him to start the blog.

Care recipients with high medical needs may require care that doesn't fit neatly into these broad divisions. One of these is administrative care: wrangling insurance companies and billing departments, handling leaves of absence or disability paperwork with HR, or cutting through obscure thickets of the Social Security Administration. We don't always think of paperwork and data collection as caregiving but it is intrinsic to modern care, as memoirist Anne Boyer points out: "The word 'care' rarely calls to mind a keyboard. The work, often unwaged or poorly paid, of those who perform care . . . is what many understand to be that which is the least technological, the most affective and intuitive. 'Care' is so often understood as a mode of feeling, neighboring, as it does, love." The gendered nature of both caregiving and administration binds the two: "The work of care and the work of data exist in a kind of paradoxical simultaneity: what both hold in common is that they are done so often by women, and like all that has historically been identified as women's work, it is work that can go by unnoticed."[27]

Administrative care comes with extraordinary frustrations, as anyone who's ever tried to make sense of an Explanation of Benefits or waded through HR guidelines knows. I had to fill out all of the paperwork for my husband's disability claims and eventual disability retirement, which involved long calls with benefits coordinators and bureaucrats. And I had it easy: Brad was a tenured, unionized professor at a public university, where the HR personnel were trying their hardest to get us everything we were entitled to. Those dealing with stingy corporations or unstable employment often endure grave frustration for little or no reward. Research and coordination of care is another aspect of this type of care: on average, caregivers spend thirteen hours a month "researching care services or information on disease, coordinating physician visits or managing financial matters." More than 60 percent of caregivers report spending significant time communicating with healthcare providers and adjusting the patient's care, and 50 percent say they act as an advocate.[28]

A particularly challenging type of care is higher-level nursing tasks, as I found after Brad's discharges. According to the Family Caregivers Alliance, 46 percent of caregivers providing "complex chronic care" (ongoing high-demand caregiving) "perform medical and nursing tasks."[29] Moreover, a majority felt they had no choice because nobody else would do it and/or insurance wouldn't pay for professional assistance.

Such nursing care is a subset of Glenn's category of direct physical care but with the painful twist of a steep learning curve—one I experienced myself, as described in preceding chapters. Just as I was hastily trained and nervous about my role in giving IV antibiotics and hooking up Brad's IV nutrition, many thousands of reluctant family members are conscripted into administering medical tasks such as wound care, giving injections, and colostomy care at home.[30]

It's easy to see how burnout can result from such overreliance on a single caregiver, and I am convinced it was a factor in mine. It's well known that healthcare workers can suffer "compassion fatigue" and desensitization to suffering because of the extreme demands of their work. I believe the high emotional demands of caring for a suffering loved one can lead to a similar kind of fatigue. On high alert and in an extreme emotional state for months, after a time I had difficulty accessing my love and compassion for my husband.

For me, part of the task at hand was sometimes trying to make sure the physician or nurse remembered: person first, cancer patient second. I reminded them of our home life, of the unique web of circumstances making a certain treatment challenging or easy. For instance, we lived close to the Cancer Center so could get there fast, but appointments at 8 a.m. or 3 p.m. were terrible because we had school-age children. They can't remember such details for every patient. But I insisted we were still people with needs, not numbers in the system's database. Reminding medical personnel of this felt like carving out an incremental, tiny space for patients—not just Brad and me, but future patients and caregivers, too—to assert needs beyond the medical.

BURNOUT DANGER: VERY HIGH

In the years to come, the heavy demands of unpaid caregiving are set to collide with the rising demographic shortage of family caregivers that I discussed in the introduction. A closer look at the numbers reveals how dire the shortage really is. In 2010 the ratio of potential caregivers (aged forty-five to sixty-four) to every individual aged eighty and up was seven to one.[31] By 2050, one study predicted, that "caregiver support ratio" will have fallen to three to one.

As signaled by the rising number of millennial caregivers, a lack of available family caregivers has spillover effects. Frail older adults rarely stop needing care, except in the sad event of their death—an event that can be hastened by inadequate care. If there is a paucity of available family members of typical caregiving age, younger people will have to step in to take their place, or else those who need care will have to seek it in institutions or from hired personnel. Moreover, as hospital costs increase and physicians come under pressure to discharge fragile patients, they may send home more patients with extreme needs like Brad's.

CAREGIVING AT THE EXTREMES

Certainly not all caregiving leads to burnout and I'm sure there are many more patient caregivers out there than I. Tracy Grant, in her 2016 essay for the *Washington Post*, says caregiving for her dying husband was the best seven months of her life.[32] And, unfortunately, there are worse ones out there, too, those whose anger or resentment has overwhelmed them. I did sometimes resent Brad, to my shame, and sometimes I was angry at him, but I tried always to think of him as a loved person—my husband, my kids' father—rather than as a burden. One of the critical elements of responsible, compassionate caregiving is keeping firmly in mind the full, coequal humanity of one's charge.

Unfortunately, our culture's narrative around disability and illness sometimes runs counter to that need. People with disabilities are often treated as less than fully human, as the brutal history of institutionalization, mistreatment, and even murder—often miscalled mercy killing—shows.[33] Often, narratives around such abuse and killing have functioned as justifications, on the grounds of caregiver stress or overwhelm. Or—as in the case of a widely reported 2019 murder-suicide of Alzheimer's patient Alma Shaver by her husband, Richard—such crimes have been framed as acts of love or ending the loved one's suffering. Writer and disability advocate Sara Luterman gives a sharp corrective to such framings in a valuable *Washington Post* piece, written in response to the latter case: "No amount of difficulty justifies the taking of a life."[34]

The overwhelm that can come with caregiving can go very bad indeed, and I want to be clear that burnout can never be an excuse for the kind of extreme bad-caregiving tales that have been played for sensationalism in thrillers. The movie *Misery* (based on a Stephen King book), in which Kathy Bates plays Annie Wilkes, a superfan who terrorizes the injured author she's supposed to be caring for, comes to mind. So does *What Ever Happened to Baby Jane?*, the famed Bette Davis and Joan Crawford film in which a former child star torments her paraplegic sister.

One of the most notorious forms of abusive caregiving is Munchausen syndrome by proxy (MSP), a rare mental illness in which caregivers fake and even exacerbate the symptoms of their charges. (The condition has been renamed factitious disorder imposed on another, or FDIA, but remains best known by its previous name.) MSP seems like a twisted expression of the martyrdom of caregiving, a desperate grab at the bittersweet pleasure of being needed. Because of the case of Gypsy Rose Blanchard, recently dramatized in the television series *The Act*, this disorder has received significant recent media attention. Often, caregivers with MSP have themselves been the victims of significant past trauma, as in the case of the mother of Julie Gregory, whose memoir *Sickened* provides a devastating look at growing up under such conditions.[35]

BURNOUT SOLUTIONS

As I discovered, it can be a challenge to find relief once you've entered a state of burnout. For many, it feels impossible. On CaregiverStress.com, comments on a post about breaking out of isolation give a sad glimpse of the realities for many caregivers. "Judy" writes: "Totally dependent no help from family, friends seem to shy away slowly, so I'm on my own. Love keeps me strong, can't afford any respite care at this time so the only time I go out alone is food shopping and then it's a rush to get back and hope all is well." A commenter named Sandy writes, "I used to go play bingo once a month, then once every two months. Now I can't remember the last time I've gone. Over several months at least. I get depressed, but I hold it in. It isn't poor Tom's fault, It's that damn Parkinson's Disease. I feel like I'm SCREAMING inside, but I put a smile on my face and go on." "Kayo" reports they've had only 48 hours off in nine years. Another woman, Claudia, has placed her husband in an Alzheimer's facility and is advised not to visit for a week; she says she doesn't know what to do to enjoy herself anymore.[36] These short online comments generated little dialogue but they hint at one option for combatting isolation: virtual communities. I've noticed that just about any article on caregiving attracts hundreds of comments from isolated, often desperate caregivers.

All these feelings can have serious health consequences, as a *New York Times* article on caregiver isolation points out, leading to depression, anxiety, and even heart attack and stroke.[37] Estimates of depression rates among caregivers are high, ranging from 40 to 70 percent.[38] Refreshingly, the *Times* piece, written by Paula Span, offers suggestions that don't put the onus back on caregivers: "It's too easy to let caregiving friends slip off our radar with a general call-if-you-need-anything," writes Span, who goes on to suggest that friends "ask . . . what would be helpful, making a list of specific tasks and parceling out assignments."[39]

Another promising option is caregiving networks, in which no one person has primary responsibility, easing the onus on any single caregiver while also reducing isolation. I've read accounts recently of younger people, especially stepping up as a group to help an ill friend who is far from family and has no obvious primary caregiver. Briallen Hopper, in her essays "Young Adult Cancer Story" and "Coasting," tells the story of how she and three others banded together as a caregiving group when their friend Ash went through cancer treatment. (Both essays are in Hopper's book *Hard to Love*.) Interestingly, none of the people in the group were especially close before the cancer diagnosis. They bonded around the rituals of caring, an endless email thread, online spreadsheets, writing together during Ash's chemo infusions, and—interestingly—reading and discussing *The Fault in Our Stars*, John Green's blockbuster young-adult novel about a girl with stage IV cancer. As Hopper describes it, "Countless people were part of Ash's many overlapping circles of care," but "over the long haul" the quartet "tended to function as a care-team core, stitched together by text and email threads."[40]

Hopper's account makes it clear that while caregiving can produce trauma in relationships—one member of the caregiving team, Sarah, saved all of their email threads but finds them too hard to revisit—it can also engender closeness and a sense of purpose. This becomes evident in the relationship that grows between Ash and care team member Lisa: "Ash and Lisa are fully family now," Hopper writes. "Before cancer, they often fit their friendship into the corner of their overscheduled lives, but in the midst of cancer, their relationship became central and essential." Hopper had a similar experience: "Ash and I have an intimacy that was precipitated by illness. It's awful to admit that we owe our current closeness to cancer, but it is almost certainly true."[41]

One tip seems to recur on every list for caregivers: attend a support group or meet with people going through something similar. The problem is that overextended caregivers can rarely meet up in the real world. Many of us have turned to online communities to alleviate the loneliness. Among these I wanted to choose carefully. Surprisingly, for me the best place was Twitter, where I was relatively anonymous. Twitter is mostly a sinkhole of bad opinions but it has welcoming corners that for me were a lifeline. Until Brad got sick I was active on Facebook, posting in my usual voice: wry observations, the occasional cynical take, kid pictures. After Brad's illness turned serious, I felt uncomfortable sharing anything but a heavily edited version of my real thoughts on caregiving. Too many friends and family members were watching my timeline for news on Brad. My own concerns would have upset people—especially if I sounded frustrated, cynical, or, worst of all, sardonic. Humor, dark humor especially, is missing from the pious public discourse around caregiving, but for me it is and was an essential coping mechanism. Janet Kim, communications director for the nonprofit advocacy group Caring Across Generations, told me that her organization has begun to highlight humor in its campaigns around caregiving, to humanize it and break the stigma. They've even partnered with the improv group Second City to do role-playing, trainings, and focus groups.[42]

Unlike Facebook, Twitter responds well to dark comedy and is unshockable. It's also full of compassionate people and a small, flickering community of honest caregivers, and even people going through stem cell transplant. There, I could post daily observations (including my photos of odd hospital art), talk about movies and TV, comment on politics, complain about caregiving, lament Brad's illness. In short, I could be myself, and I could almost always get a fave or two out of it. Within the world's biggest stew of anonymity and contention, somehow, I felt like I could be seen, and some of the connections I made with others in similar situations grew into deep (albeit long-distance) friendships.

Connecting with others, taking respites where possible, and finding physical ways to de-stress are part of the science-based recommendations in Emily and Amelia Nagoski's book, previously discussed in the introduction. Addressed explicitly to women, *Burnout* proposes moving through the stress response and negative emotions via exercise, action, and conscious reframing of our roles.[43] I was particularly intrigued by their call to direct action against the larger systems that trap all of us and I found it a potentially valuable resource for anyone who feels burned out by the demands placed upon them.

One of the things I did, during my worst days, was write. Sometimes it was the word-processing equivalent of a scribble, my ranting protestations against what was happening in my life. Sometimes I tried to put together something a little more eloquent. When Brad was in the hospital, sometimes I had my laptop with me. I maintained a (paid) membership in an online writing workshop facilitated by a dear friend. It kept alive a little bit of the spark of my work and self. As that pressured summer gave way to fall and Brad started to gain a little more strength, I hoped to return to the more formal writing work I'd dropped during the most intense phases of Brad's illness.

SIX

INVALUABLE

Work and the Economics of Caring

September came at last. The kids went back to school. Brad, having gained more independence, could navigate our house by himself and be home alone for brief periods. He'd gotten better at using the accessibility features on his phone and he could call Lyft or paratransit to get to some of his many medical appointments. I was itching to get back to some kind of work. I didn't want to be seen as "just" a caregiver anymore, my only value tied up in what I did for other people. Caring may be a rewarding vocation for many but for me it wasn't enough to feel personally and professionally satisfied. I needed to be expressing myself and living for myself, and doing that through some kind of work—paid or not—felt urgent.

I also felt like it was my turn—in fact, past time for my turn. I was turning forty-four that fall and my professional dreams had been on hold for a long time; it felt like I needed to pursue them while I still could. I thought back to the final season of *Friday Night Lights*, a show I'd rewatched while breastfeeding my younger daughter.[1] In the finale the coach's wife, Tami Taylor, gets a big job offer to become a college counselor, which would require the family to move away from Texas, where her husband has always coached football. They're fighting about it and she points out that she has moved with him, supported him, and put her own goals on hold for him: "It's my turn, babe," she says. In a flash-forward montage that ends the series, we see that she gets to follow her dream. But life isn't much like television: for starters, I'm no Tami Taylor and Brad was far from being a state-champ football coach. But for more than a decade I'd put a lot on hold for him and our family: I'd left a prominent magazine job in the Bay Area to become a freelancer in the smaller city where he had a tenure-track position. I scaled back on my work to take primary responsibility for our second baby when Brad became department chair. I dropped any semblance of a professional life to care for him when he needed me. Now, it seemed to me that his chances of working again, at least in the near future, were nil. I wanted him to support my career, to the extent that he was able. It was my turn, babe.

Looking back, I was rushing things in my impatience to change my situation. Brad wasn't really able to act as the manager of our household or even as an equal partner. His vision was slightly improved but not good enough for him to drive or read. It was unrealistic to expect that I'd go back to full-time work and I knew it, but I didn't want a high-powered career in any case; I wanted to be able to write longer projects, such as this book, which was slowly starting to take shape in my mind. I wanted to at least lay the groundwork for a shift in our family dynamics—to give notice that I would need my work and career to take priority as he continued to recover. But Brad had other ideas.

TUG OF WAR

While Brad was at his sickest I had done occasional tasks connected with his professional life: checking emails, returning some library books, going to campus at the start of each term to update the sign on his office door saying he was on medical leave that semester. I'd also been in touch, frequently, with Human Resources about his benefits and leave. In part thanks to the oddities of the academic calendar, which meant that he didn't need to use sick time in summer, Brad's sick leave extended far longer than most. Although I didn't exactly enjoy handling such administrative matters, securing his benefits was obviously important for our whole family, as our health insurance came through his job. But I drew the line at helping him with his more creative endeavors.

Back when Brad was well he used to joke that he would, someday, appoint me his literary executrix. He said it would fall to me, after his death, to edit his poetry collections, to arrange his papers, to publish his archive. I laughed and never agreed, but I never refused either. When his death no longer seemed a far-distant event but a real possibility, he stopped making this joke. I quietly declined to help him with submitting poems and a manuscript when he was blind and unable to do it himself; I wanted precious time to write for myself, but more often that time went to running our household.

Throughout the summer Brad had been working on poems about his illness, written by dictation, as well as an academic project he'd started long before he got sick. When his mother was still in Sacramento she acted as his amanuensis, helping him submit poems to journals and, later, a full manuscript to presses. (The manuscript has since been published as a book titled *The Scars, Aligned.*)[2] After she went home to Canada, Brad hired a graduate student from his former department to help with his research and writing. They frequently sat in the living room working, where I could hear them as I paid bills or tidied the house.

I was terribly, angrily envious of Brad then—not of his illness, of course, but of the fact that he had time to work on his writing and I didn't. Hiring a paid assistant for Brad seemed to me, in my burned-out state, symbolically to underscore the greater value of Brad's creative work over mine. At the same time, fairly or not, I wasn't sure I wanted to support his work. I was all too painfully aware that his mental clarity and sharpness weren't what they had been before he got sick. Looking back, I cringe at how much I doubted the value of his work, but a conflict we'd had while he was still in the hospital—and which dragged on for months—was contributing to my harsh judgment.

When Brad's eyes were sewn shut in the spring, he had asked me for a voice recorder. I brought in one I had always used for interviews for articles I was writing; since I was no longer working, I had no need for it. He dictated into it for hours, giving a rambling and graphic account of his hospital experience, and asked me to transcribe it. I was short on time to accomplish even basic tasks and I refused. I did finally send it to a transcriptionist I've used for interviews, paying a dollar a minute. The transcription ran more than twenty pages, single spaced, and Brad asked me if I would edit it into a sort of Day in the Life journal. He wanted me to post the result on the blog we were keeping about his cancer and treatment. Reluctantly, I started on it, but got no farther than the first wordy, confused page, consumed with vicarious embarrassment. He was heavily medicated when he made the recordings and a lot of them didn't make sense. I quietly failed to make time to edit it and hoped he would forget all about it. In the summer, though, he asked again. I felt I was protecting him from his own lack of mental clarity—the voice on the page sounded nothing like his writing, which I know nearly as well as I know my own—but in truth I was also protecting myself. I couldn't bear to wade through his murky ordeal again; I was already forced to see it, and its fallout, every day.

I put him off several times and finally confessed that I wasn't willing to spend the time—that I didn't think the transcript had any value. Was I wrong not to do what he asked of me? I thought again of *Middlemarch*: as Casaubon gets sicker he demands that Dorothea carry forward his work if he should die. He spends hours explaining to his young wife the principles he wishes to use in completing the scholarly work she knows to be worthless. She fears he may force a promise from her to edit and compile those "mixed heaps of material."[3]

Dorothea's description of Casaubon's papers reminded me not just of Brad's transcript but of certain bags that sat for years in our garage. They were ordinary grocery bags, stuffed with crumpled, illegible scraps, some inside second layers of plastic bags. They were Brad's: drafts of his poems, some scrawled on the endpapers of books and torn out, some written on fading receipts. He'd had them shipped from his childhood home in Canada to California nearly twenty years ago and hadn't looked at them since. But there they were.

Dorothea questions her own judgment and what she owes to her husband, living or dead. She has come to dislike him during their marriage, which has been fraught with unhappy, understated conflict. She nevertheless does her duty by him conscientiously, even tenderly. She cares for him, wraps him in a blanket, is solicitous at all times, hides her impatience. But she has a rebellious spirit and a strong will underneath it all and she balks at promising undying loyalty to his will after death. Over the course of her disappointing marriage Dorothea has already sacrificed a considerable number of her ambitions.

Dorothea is as unselfish as my mother-in-law was in helping Brad prepare his manuscript for submission, but the integrity of Dorothea's character makes it all but impossible for her to take on work she doesn't believe in. After agonized inner debate, however, she decides she will promise Casaubon to do whatever he asks, including finishing his book, after his death, even though she knows she will be miserable: "Neither law nor the world's opinion compelled her to this—only her husband's nature and her own compassion, only the ideal and not the real yoke of marriage. She saw clearly enough the whole situation, yet she was fettered: she could not smite the stricken soul that entreated hers."[4] This, in a nutshell, is the trap of caregiving: I've felt bound by both love and old-fashioned duty to carry out the wishes of the ill person for whom I care. But I am not a Victorian woman trained to decades of self-denial. I couldn't take on such a life at the cost of my whole self.

THE ECONOMIC PENALTY OF CARING

I can't imagine how I could have made time to work at a paid job during the worst of Brad's illness but I was fortunate to have the luxury of not doing so. Many caregivers must continue working to put food on the table—often at the cost of their sleep and health—and most take a far more damaging financial hit than I did. As Evelyn Glenn writes, "The demands of intensive care leave caregivers with little time or energy to look after their own wellbeing, so that their own health suffers"; moreover, a majority of women caregivers adjust their work schedules to accommodate caregiving, retire early, or quit their jobs.[5]

I've been a freelance writer for more than fifteen years. Throughout my career my earnings have varied tremendously, but previously, in a good year, I could expect to make in the mid five figures. During the two years that Brad's illness was at its height, I took no more than a couple of assignments, and my writing income dropped to less than a couple thousand dollars per year. I estimate my lost pay at somewhere in the neighborhood of $80,000, though it's impossible to put an exact figure on it. There were, of course, other hits to my finances as well: dipping into savings to pay for in-home care and paying extra to have groceries delivered, laundry sent out, and children cared for. And then there were longer-term, hidden opportunity costs: when I quit pitching articles, I lost contact with editors who used to send me regular assignments. I've gone back to work but my income hasn't recovered—though that's in part a function of my own choice to focus on different aspects of my career, including writing about caregiving.

The real question is not how my family could afford care, but how anyone in the US can bear the economic burden of caregiving. Examples of the challenges abound in real life and in fictitious representations, where economic questions quietly underpin the hard choices that characters must make. In Rachel Khong's recent darkly comic novel *Goodbye, Vitamin*, for instance, narrator Ruth Young must quit her job in San Francisco, move home to southern California, and help care for her father, whose worsening dementia has forced him to retire early.[6] The narrative softens the harsh financial circumstances with quirky humor, as when Ruth dreams that she has the Midas touch, but instead of gold everything turns to aluminum, now banned from the family home because of its connection with Alzheimer's.

In Viet Thanh Nguyen's short story "I'd Love You to Want Me," published in his collection *The Refugees*, the aging Professor Khanh has dementia. His wife, named only as Mrs. Khanh, is reluctant to admit he needs full-time care. A power struggle ensues between Mrs. Khanh and their first-generation American son over who must sacrifice their work to care for the patriarch. The rewards of Mrs. Khanh's job at a library reference desk aren't purely financial: "Answering those questions, Mrs. Khanh always felt the gratification that made her job worthwhile, the pleasure of being needed."[7] She doesn't find the same pleasure in being needed by her husband, underscoring how the financial aspects of caregiving are bound up in questions of love and duty.

We even see this struggle in as beloved a text as Louisa May Alcott's *Little Women*, in which the perpetually broke March family must borrow money for Mrs. March to go to Washington, DC, to care for her husband, stricken ill while serving as a Union Army chaplain in the Civil War. They borrow from their usual source: rich Aunt March, for whom daughter Jo works as a companion. The money comes, as usual, with strings attached. The price is a lecture: "Everything was arranged by the time Laurie returned with a note from Aunt March, enclosing the desired sum, and a few lines repeating what she had often said before, that she had always told them it was absurd for March to go into the army, always predicted that no good would come of it, and she hoped they would take her advice the next time. Mrs. March put the note in the fire, the money in her purse, and went on with her preparations."[8] This leads to perhaps the best-known financial caregiving sacrifice in literature: Jo March selling her hair (her "one beauty") for $25.

Contemporary family caregivers take an enormous economic hit for their work. According to the joint AARP and National Alliance for Caregiving 2009 report *Caregiving in the United States*, 70 percent of caregivers have cut back on work hours, left the workforce, taken a leave of absence, or shifted to a less demanding job—and female caregivers make these economically punishing choices at a higher rate than men. Such financial sacrifices are also, for obvious reasons, a disproportionate hardship for lower-income families.[9] According to Gail Sheehy's *Passages in Caregiving*, perhaps the most helpful practical guide on the market, one in six family caregivers lost a job during the recession that began in 2008.[10] That figure, large as it is, doesn't account for the thousands of others who had to quit jobs or reduce hours to accommodate caregiving.

The enormous economic impact of the 2020 coronavirus pandemic further exposes the costs of caring for society's most vulnerable. The pandemic had a severe economic impact on women, especially women of color, who suffered job losses at an alarming rate, often because of the pressures of providing care for children and other family members. As the pandemic wore on, its effects on working women became so extreme that a report by the nonprofit newsroom *The 19th* called it, simply, "America's First Female Recession," noting that the pandemic accelerated female job loss, often because of the challenges of providing care: "When the economy crumbled, women fell—hard."[11]

The caregiving penalty goes far beyond lost pay for reduced hours of work. It also costs us considerable money. An AARP survey figured caregivers on average spend $7,000 per year out of their pockets on associated costs.[12] Kristina Brown, a medical student at Yale and a Black woman, writes affectingly in a recent *Washington Post* piece about caring for her disabled mother as a teenager and its economic impact on her family. She also points out that those who, like herself, begin caregiving early in life may struggle to find a job that allows them flexibility for family responsibilities. "Caregiving fuels generational poverty," she writes, "disproportionately affecting millennials and women who take on that role in their families." Black caregivers take a particularly high economic hit from caregiving, as they tend to have lower household incomes than their white counterparts but spend a similar dollar amount on care costs, making those costs a higher percentage of their income (a staggering 34 percent, compared to 14 percent for white caregivers).[13]

For all, economic effects multiply over time. The less any of us caregivers participate in the workforce, the less we are able to afford health insurance of our own, and the more our economic insecurity grows. When we reach old age we're not able to collect as much in retirement income. A 2006 study showed female caregivers were about 2.5 times more likely to end up in poverty later in life than their non-caregiver counterparts. A 1999 MetLife study, cited by Evelyn Glenn, tallied up the mean lifetime financial loss from caregiving at more than half a million dollars.[14] A 2011 study calculated an average lifetime loss of $324,000 for a woman leaving the labor force early to care for a parent.[15] "Economists say the virtual absence of support for eldercare is a prime suspect explaining why the share of women taking part in the labor force stalled in the late 1990s after rising relentlessly for 50 years," reports the *New York Times* in a recent article—which summed up the problem neatly in its headline: "Why Aren't More Women Working? They're Caring for Parents."[16]

The hits on American families suffering medical crises, of course, are hardly confined to the challenges caregivers face. Unaffordable healthcare costs cause many families to lose their homes, go bankrupt, or forgo lifesaving medical care, a criminal state of affairs and a far bigger systemic problem than I can possibly address. But the cultural devaluing of our caregivers—from early childhood education to eldercare attendants—contributes enormously to the problem. As Anne-Marie Slaughter notes in *Unfinished Business*, "Not valuing caregiving is the taproot, the deeper problem that gives rise to distortion and discrimination in multiple areas of American society. When we open our eyes and change our lenses to focus on competition and care rather than women and work, we can see new solutions and new coalitions that can open the door to progress and change. Care can provide a new political banner under which all women can unite."[17]

Many forms of caring exist, all sharing some of the same challenges and demands of tending to the sick: childcare, eldercare, maintaining social ties, the (presumably) mutual care of marriage, and even volunteering or seemingly small home or work tasks, such as taking on social planning, washing up abandoned coffee cups in a shared breakroom, and writing thank-you notes. Many kinds of invisible, uncompensated work go into these critical social functions, among them care work, domestic labor, kin work, memory work, and managing mental load.

The *New York Times* recently estimated the value of such unpaid labor performed by women worldwide at nearly $10.9 trillion, noting that such work "remains largely invisible to economists"—but that people certainly notice if the supply is disrupted. And that's putting our labor at a low price. As the introduction to the interactive piece notes, "If American women earned minimum wage for the unpaid work they do around the house and caring for relatives, they would have made $1.5 trillion last year."[18] But such labor is expected for free: "Traditional expectations that caring for children, the elderly and the infirm should be done gratis within the family obscure the true economic value of this work. And yet . . . women provide a huge unacknowledged subsidy to the smooth functioning of our economies, which would grind to a halt if women stopped doing this work."[19] In addition, there's an unspoken expectation that women will perform all this work without complaint, as Slaughter points out: "Women . . . face much more cultural pressure to be caregivers, and perfect ones at that, than men do."[20]

There's no one broad term for all that gendered work, though lately "emotional labor" has started to be used as a general (and somewhat imprecise) catchall.[21] Sociologist Arlie Hochschild originally coined the phrase in her book *The Managed Heart*, to describe the work of performing or managing emotions in paid employment—such as flight attendants being always pleasant—but "emotional labor" has taken on a much larger life of its own in popular parlance. Hochschild herself gives us a possible alternative phrase for some of this gendered domestic work in the title of another one of her books, *The Second Shift*, but that specifically describes the work undertaken at home after completing paid labor. Better broad terms would be "caring labor" and "invisible labor," either of which can encompass all the things we do to care for others: sending birthday cards to distant relatives (often called kin work), picking up the house (domestic work), making Jell-O for a puking spouse (caregiving), remembering the every-other-week schedule for recycling pickup (mental load), reminding the kids to scoop the cat litter (household management, parenting), running interference on sibling squabbles (parenting), maintaining the family photo archives (memory work), and so on.

In *The Second Shift*, Hochschild clearly links the challenges around various caring tasks to the priorities of American capitalism, which has led feminism broadly to prioritize "empowerment" for women and to "sidetrack" care. Caring for others has become what she calls "a hand-me-down job," pushed from men to women, from high-income and white women to lower-income women, primarily women of color and immigrants. The "big challenge" at the center of her work—and of feminism—is how "to value and share the duties of caring for loved ones."[22]

That's a question society hasn't yet answered, as I found. Caring for my ill spouse concentrated these various forms of invisible work into one almost unbearably intense experience. American culture codes these tasks as female and women as naturally better nurturers.

THE VALUE OF CARE

The necessary work of family caregivers has enormous worth; remember that AARP estimate of the market value of unpaid care labor in at a staggering $470 billion? That figure comes from an estimated 37 billion hours of care, calculated at an hourly wage of just over $12.[23] This figure reflects an average of about sixteen hours per week spent on care. Many caregivers' roles demand far more time; mine certainly did. The healthcare system depends on this kind of care for countless vulnerable patients.

Despite the obvious value of this work there is no remuneration for most American caregivers. The time spent helping a family member is typically uncompensated by public programs or insurance, though there are states with programs offering caregivers economic support. Some families arrange to pay a family member by pooling resources. But our healthcare system and government programs do little, and in most cases nothing, to support caregivers. As Gail Sheehy (writing before passage of the Affordable Care Act) noted in her *Passages in Caregiving*: "Instead of subsidizing people who quit their jobs to take care of their loved ones, the government has slashed Medicare benefits and funding for home-health-care agencies."[24] Many agencies and insurance companies have also shifted care-related costs to families. The only benefit federally guaranteed to family caregivers—and then only to those who work for companies with more than fifty employees—is twelve weeks of unpaid leave per year via the Family and Medical Leave Act. FMLA (at which I look more closely, along with other legal resources for caregivers, in the conclusion) provides a little relief in terms of time but constitutes a de facto economic penalty for those workers who can afford to take it. Moreover, it's not available to all workers, and in any case isn't enough to meet the care needs of ongoing disability or eldercare, chronic illness, or someone suffering a major health crisis. "Our country has not yet recognized the importance of providing paid family leave," says Lynn Feinberg of AARP. "Most family caregivers who are caring for someone who's seriously ill or has a disability can't afford to stop out of the workforce without getting a paycheck."[25]

In 2020 an emergency expansion of FMLA, called FFCRA (Families First Coronavirus Response Act), required some employers to offer paid leave for coronavirus-related reasons such as self-quarantining or caring for a quarantined individual, but this expansion was temporary, lasting only to the end of the year.[26] Moreover, as Joan C. Williams—director of the Center for WorkLife Law at the University of California, Hastings, College of the Law—pointed out in an August 2020 *New York Times* op-ed primarily focused on childcare, "Figuring out whether you're eligible for Families First is so complicated that a chart explaining the program looks like a game of Chutes and Ladders." Williams reports that a spike in calls to her center's legal-resource hotline "make it clear that Families First is falling short."[27]

Even before the pandemic highlighted the need for better policies around family leave and caregiving, a few states, including California and New Jersey, were considering a caregiver tax credit to offer some relief. A $3,000 federal tax credit for caregivers, which AARP and other organizations have advocated for, failed in congressional committee in 2019.[28] Such failures, broadly speaking, are part of the deficit of empathy in America. Our undervaluing of care for the marginalized and the weak harms us all.

THE FUNHOUSE MIRROR: CARE COSTS

A critical systemic failure is our costly and cruel healthcare system: a dysfunctional patchwork of rapacious for-profit entities, overburdened nonprofits, and an inadequate social safety net. Healthcare is an enormous sector of the economy, accounting for 17.7 percent of the gross domestic product ($3.6 trillion) in 2018.[29] I view the way our system ties healthcare access to one's job as a moral outrage and favor a form of universal healthcare. (I write more about policy solutions around healthcare and caregiving in the conclusion.)

Though it has always been expensive to care for the sick, in the US today the relationship between healthcare and its market value is uniquely irrational. Hospital services for emergencies are wildly expensive; home care for recovery or chronic illness is underpaid or worth nothing at all.

At some point in the middle of 2016 I started receiving long-delayed Explanation of Benefits in thick envelopes from our insurer. Here are the figures I saw when I opened them:

$1,085,933.82

$1,091,127.76

$3,922,498.67

The total—more than $6 million—was eye-popping.[30] The biggest figures were for room and board; I joked that because Brad wasn't eating anything by mouth for a good ten weeks of his hospitalization, they should have given him a discount on the board. In total that year I received 209 Explanation of Benefits notices—more than one every other day. Each was a reminder of how medical costs are obsessively enumerated. Every IV bag, every brief hospital bedside chat with a specialist, every shot of insulin has a billing code and a dollar figure, usually large, attached to it. Insurers rarely if ever pay that full amount, instead paying what's called a negotiated rate differential; in fact, the full billed amounts on such EOBs are inadmissible in California courts as proof of costs associated with illness. They are a fantasy of cost, unrelated to the actual value of care.[31]

We paid nothing for all that care, shown on the EOBs as being worth millions of dollars. Our insurance company, Blue Shield, contracted with UC Davis Medical Center to pay a much lower flat rate for stem cell transplants. Blue Shield won't disclose its contracted flat-fee rate for a stem cell transplant at the Center. I recall, however, a flat-fee figure on those Explanation of Benefits notices: the number stuck in my head is $25,000 to cover 150 days of hospitalization. It may well have been more, but even ten times that figure is nowhere near the $6 million in bills generated for Brad's hospitalization.

Still, how could anyone look those EOBs in the face and not blanch a little? If we hadn't had the kind of insurance we did, bills of this kind would have devastated us.

Medical costs are something like a funhouse mirror, reflecting vast or tiny sums with little apparent relationship to actual value. Come to think of it, funhouse mirrors always made me feel a little woozy, like those figures. If the relationship between medical bills and the value of care seems distorted, however, that's nothing compared to the relationship between the value of caregiving and how little most caregivers are paid. Most paid care workers make subsistence-level wages. And as we've seen, the answer for most family caregivers is nothing.

REVALUING CARE

How did we come to a point where caring for our loved ones—an activity that provides some $470 billion of uncompensated value to a $3.6 trillion sector of the economy—is not considered an economic activity or even included in the GDP?[32] The answer may lie in the historical shift to an industrialized economy, in which women were—ideologically speaking, at least—transformed from economic actors in a household to dependents. In preindustrial times, Evelyn Glenn writes, care work was part of a home-based economic system, and both men and women were understood as economic actors who contributed to the household: "Women were primarily responsible for caring, but they also contributed to the family's livelihood by producing goods for family consumption and for barter and for cash. . . . A wife's unpaid labor was commonly understood to have economic value."[33] Prior to the Industrial Revolution, and in agrarian households, men's labor also often didn't result in cash income, but rather in the production of barterable or consumable goods.

The industrialization of the late eighteenth and early nineteenth centuries, which meant a move from cottage industries and farm labor to jobs outside the home, broadly divided the public and private spheres. Thus for elites and the broad middle classes, the home became separate from—indeed a retreat from—professional life; the workplace was part of the public, economic sphere. The latter was the realm of men, the former that of women. There were many exceptions to this ideal, particularly among the working class, people of color, and immigrant groups, where many women worked—including in the homes of those elites, and in the historical case of Black women, by force as enslaved labor.

The broad outlines, however, of this shift meant that, as Glenn writes, "the concept of a family made up of a male earner employed outside the home and wife/mother engaged in unpaid reproductive labor at home became the dominant ideal."[34] The shift also came along with an idealization and sentimentalization of such women's work, something we see in the Victorian ideal of the Angel in the House. Caregiving, among other types of so-called women's work, was considered a natural vocation of women, not something that could be counted in the economic realm. As Glenn points out, Western culture has long defined the caring performed by a spouse, daughter, or mother as a moral duty rather than an economic activity: "Importantly . . . as embodied in the law and in everyday understandings, these unpaid [caring] responsibilities were stripped of economic significance and instead viewed as moral and spiritual vocations."[35]

This work, however, was far from easy—or solely spiritual: "The private household caring of middle-class and elite women was valorized and privileged," Glenn writes. "Yet, there was a fundamental contradiction between the spiritual qualities attributed to the ideal wife/mother and the heavy physical labor that was involved in caring."[36] Nursing the sick was hard, unpleasant work: tending wounds, emptying bedpans, and physically moving sick bodies. In real life, Louisa May Alcott was "the nurse in the family" for the Alcotts, including for her sister Lizzie (the model for Beth in *Little Women*). She glosses over the harsher realities of caregiving in *Little Women*, written as it was for children, but an earlier work, *Hospital Sketches*, paints a vivid picture of the grueling nature of nineteenth-century nursing: "My three days' experiences had begun with a death, and . . . a somewhat abrupt plunge into the superintendence of a ward containing forty beds, where I spent my shining hours washing faces, serving rations, giving medicine, and sitting in a very hard chair, with pneumonia on one side, diphtheria on the other, five typhoids on the opposite, and a dozen dilapidated patriots, hopping, lying, and lounging about. "[37]

Such heavy labor was even heavier and harder for those forced to engage in it, namely, the enslaved Black people in the American South—which further contributed to the stigma attached to such work.[38] Enslaved Black women, especially those too old for hard physical labor, were often forced into caregiving roles for both white enslavers and fellow enslaved people. Interestingly, Glenn notes, some enslaved women were able to use their power as healers to subvert the order of the plantation, caring for their families and community members and fostering bonds of love and compassion that the masters tried to break. In addition, many enslaved "nurses" were able to use effective remedies based on their knowledge of herb lore, protesting against white doctors' ineffectual treatments, such as calomel.[39] The multiple ways in which these enslaved women were oppressed—through their blackness, their slave status, their gender—all contributed to the devaluation of not only the care they provided but their skill as healers. Ai-jen Poo writes,

> As well as being associated with the unpaid work of slaves, and then the poorly paid work of African Americans and immigrants, caregiving is and has always been associated with women, alongside other unpaid work in the home. Such skills and labor from women "simply have not been counted within our economy's measures of productivity. . . . It has just been assumed that women will perform them.[40]

The idea of separate spheres might sound like a relic of the Victorian age but author Alissa Quart, writing about the present-day challenges of the middle class in her book *Squeezed*, shows how this framework has subtly persisted—and continues to keep workers who care for others from being properly paid: "It's as if we Americans assume that when people spend their time loving or tending to others they have somehow stepped out of the commercial—and thus any pragmatic, valuable, and intelligent—sphere. . . . Low pay and lack of respect are, in a sense, what they earn for having jobs taking care of America's most vulnerable."[41] As Poo points out in *The Age of Dignity*, "Our major laws and systems for care are based on standards and demographics from another era."[42] Moreover, I'd add, even in that semi-mythical era, women's domesticity was already an idealized fiction, one mainly relevant to middle-class and wealthy white society. Such a fiction allowed these privileged women to overlook their reliance on the work of women of lower socioeconomic status.

The professionalization of medical knowledge, and the corresponding rise of institutions and hospitals in the late nineteenth and early twentieth centuries, led doctors and nurses to denigrate nonprofessional care as unscientific. A similar process happened in the history of obstetrics, where the traditional knowledge of midwives—often women of color or otherwise marginalized women—was pushed aside. Home births became seen as dangerous. In many states, midwifery was outright banned. Home nursing care was not treated quite so harshly, but according to Glenn, in the nineteenth and early twentieth centuries, physicians increasingly disparaged family caregivers, saying that they coddled patients and advocating strenuously for more hospitalization: "Wives and mothers continued to provide home nursing, but their work became less autonomous because it was ideally to be carried out under a physician's direction."[43] In effect, that shift demoted family caregivers to lower status—further devaluing their work.

There's a deep stigma still attached to care work. Quart looks at the economic pressures on American families (though not directly at caregiving for the ill), tracing how care work gets sidelined. In a chapter on "extreme day care" (which runs round the clock for night and swing-shift workers), Quart meditates on the "contempt" she sees expressed for care work, noting its "roots in everything from religion to American notions of what comprises achievement. The historic origins of this contempt: care work has long been associated with charity and piety. Care workers were either not paid or paid in alms." The refusal to value care work is the flip side of lofty rhetoric about its pricelessness: "Regular salaries would defeat the longstanding spiritual valence of care work as self-sacrifice for others," Quart writes.[44]

In *Creating Capabilities*, philosopher Martha Nussbaum calls for "a great human investment in care" as an alternative to traditional development theory, which prioritizes building economies.[45] "Currently, a good deal of this work is being done by women, and much of it without pay, as if it were the natural result of love," Nussbaum notes. Care work, she argues, is a direct cause of gender inequality: "Women are handicapped in other areas of life by the work they are doing in the home."[46] Nussbaum relates this phenomenon to present-day notions of masculinity that view caring tasks as "unmanly."

In a pragmatic approach, University of British Columbia psychology professor Toni Schmader has suggested repositioning the caring professions with new terminology, as psychologist and author Darcy Lockman details in her recent book *All the Rage: Mothers, Fathers, and the Myth of*

Equal Partnership. Schmader has suggested an acronym analogous to STEM (science, technology, engineering, and math): HEED, which designates careers in healthcare, elementary education, and the domestic sphere. Unfortunately, Schmader found men resistant to valuing HEED careers as equal to those in STEM. "Therein lies the problem with our biases," Lockman writes: "Men see nothing to gain in becoming more like women."[47]

It takes a mental shift to buck all the conventional wisdom of what it means to care for others. After all, in sickness and in health is even written into marriage vows, and the idea that women, especially, owe free care to others runs deep. I've seen caregivers argue that being paid would actually cheapen or corrupt their emotional attachment to the person they care for. Bullshit, I say. That argument consigns us all to the draining, fruitless self-sacrifice that props up the current system, enriching its overlords at the expense of struggling individuals—mostly women—who deserve better.

In *The Age of Dignity*, Ai-jen Poo contends that care work does have intrinsic value—offering the opportunity to learn from and form relationships with our elders—but she also argues it must have economic value. She approaches the value of care not with sentimentality but with thoughtful compassion for both care recipients and providers: "The more we recognize the value of seniors, people with disabilities, and others who build rich and satisfying lives through extended networks of personal assistance and care, the more skilled we will become at structuring interdependence into our everyday lives."[48] Poo doesn't leave it at that; her activism aims at building broader social support for care networks to relieve the strain on individual family caregivers. For her the critical shift needs also to come through social change and government policies to support meaningful caregiving in practical ways—giving caregiving the valuation it deserves. Such a shift, she suggests, would enrich us all.

In *Unfinished Business*, Slaughter points out that "both women and men who experience the dual tug of care and career and as a result must make compromises at work pay a price." Because caregiving (which, in Slaughter's work, includes childcare) is so deeply gendered, it's often seen as a problem only for women, when, as Slaughter argues, it's a larger social issue: "Redefining the women's problem as a care problem thus broadens our lens and allows us to focus much more precisely on the real issue: the undervaluing of care, no matter who does it."[49] I look at policy proposals and solutions to support caregivers in the conclusion, but I believe it's critical to erase the stigma around care work. We must move toward seeing it as a valuable social effort rather than a draining, private individual obligation. But it's not easy to make that shift even on an individual level. I know only too well how the feeling of being worth less when I'm "just" caregiving instead of writing or pursuing more economically productive goals. After all, that's why I wanted to get back to work.

ZERO-SUM GAME

In principle, as summer turned to fall, Brad agreed that it would be my turn. As he improved, he promised, he would support me in returning to work. But then he also started talking about going back to teaching himself. I was aghast. Not only was he extremely immune suppressed but he was also severely visually impaired, unadept at adaptive technology, and receiving frequent treatments. His energy levels were limited and unpredictable; sometimes he needed to rest nearly the whole day. If he went back to teaching even half time, I argued, I would still be handling everything and then some at home and supporting his wish to teach in the bargain.

His interest in returning to teaching was spurred by more than a little wishful thinking (in truth, so was my thought that I could start spending significant amounts of time writing again), but also by an impending deadline with his long-term leave. We'd learned that in February 2017 he would run out of disability leave. In order to keep receiving benefits he would need to either return to work a minimum of half time or take a disability retirement. At the time he was forty-six and I don't think he liked the thought of being retired and ending his career so young. But then again I was two years younger and I hadn't planned on ending my career either.

What our conversations—okay, fights—revealed to me was how little he really thought about all the invisible work I did to create the conditions of our lives—his life—and how thoroughly he assumed I would just keep doing it. It didn't enter his head that if he went back to teaching, all the work of home would default back to me. The labor I did was beyond invisible to him; he couldn't even comprehend its existence when I tried to explain it.

It was hard to tell him, as well, that I honestly didn't think he could handle teaching. I gave my reasons: his suppressed immune system, his learning curve with adaptive technology. He argued that the disability center on campus would support him with the technology and he would hire readers and assistants; I argued that everything, from grading papers to planning lectures, would be orders of magnitude more time consuming and thus a greater drain on his limited energy. A lot of my argument, though, boiled down to the same one Tami Taylor made: What about me? Isn't it my turn? He finally conceded that it was—and that his returning to work would pose a major challenge, one that would be untenable for me and our family. He agreed to take the retirement and that, at least in principle, he would be working toward supporting my career and taking on more of the labor of home. I began filling out his disability retirement paperwork. I felt optimistic about the future for the first time in a long time and I booked a trip to Mexico for a solo writing retreat later that fall.

I booked that trip with a departure on November 9, 2016—the morning after Election Day. At the time I felt optimistic about that too. It turned out that nothing would go as I had hoped. Our argument about who would get to go back to work proved moot. A new diagnosis—another thing we'd never heard of—derailed his recovery, leading me to a fresh reckoning with how to balance the responsibilities of caregiving.

SEVEN

A LACK OF REASONABLE OPTIONS

Sandwiched Caregiving

In late September 2016, at the height of our wrangling over work and family, came a call from Brad's nurse coordinator. He needed a PET scan, urgently. A suspicious new virus had popped up in his blood tests: Epstein-Barr, best known for causing mononucleosis. We hadn't known they were testing for that and had no idea what the implications were, but neither one of us liked the sound of needing a PET scan. He'd just had one a few weeks before and it had been clear.

We were right to worry. The new scan showed tumors in his liver, lungs, spine, and abdominal cavity. It was a widespread new lymphoma, the doctor explained, a rare complication of his post-transplant immune suppression. Brad's immune suppression had allowed Epstein-Barr virus to flourish and his depleted T-cells couldn't fight it effectively, so his B-cells—previously normal—were making a futile attempt to do so. As they proliferated they became the tumors of a life-threatening cancer.

This news came as a further shock. I'd been worrying about a relapse of his original cancer or flares of GvHD or an opportunistic infection, but we'd never heard of a complication like this. Dr. T estimated that, with treatment, Brad might have a year to live. Exhausted already, I braced for the onslaught of a new decline. And I worried about the kids. They had already been through so much. They'd missed their dad for months while he was in the hospital and had seen him come home completely different from the father they knew. I'd adjusted our family habits and changed their birthday parties and put them into aftercare to accommodate caring for Brad. I knew, also, that I hadn't given them all the mothering I would have liked to. They were doing pretty well on the whole—remarkably so given the disruptions they'd seen over the previous two years—but the thought of preparing them for their father's death, just when we'd all gotten some hope back, made my stomach clench. I pushed away the thought of what it would be like to raise them as a widow; it was too much just to consider shepherding them through Brad's presumed decline.

I thought about all that would be required over the following months: the need to support him, to talk to doctors, to set up the house for a protracted illness, possibly to set up hospice care. I asked Brad about what kind of death he wanted and tried to figure out how I would help him have a good one. I told him that if he were to die I would keep his memory alive for our girls. They would remember him, I swore. I would take them to Canada to see his family. I would, as ever, be indomitable.

I wasn't sure whether I even meant all those promises, but for his sake and for our girls I made them anyway. I felt like I was living that glib truism "fake it till you make it." I'd felt like I'd been faking it for months—years, even—but maybe it didn't matter as long as I kept things going. Or maybe it was my best self and my long love for Brad—which had faded from my view by that time—rising up in the crisis. Brad looked straight at me, even though his clouded blue eyes couldn't see well enough to recognize the pain on my face.

"Don't make too many promises," said my husband. "You don't know if you can keep them."

EMOTIONAL TWISTER

When I promised Brad I would take care of our children if he died, it went without saying I was already doing so. As his illness continued I began both consciously and unconsciously to prioritize care for our daughters, whose fleeting childhood wouldn't wait for their dad's illness. The conflict between oneself and one's care recipient becomes even more complex when we introduce the competing needs of others. If caring for my husband and preserving my sense of self sometimes felt like a zero-sum game, as discussed in the preceding chapter, factoring in the needs of our children raised the stakes.

Almost every caregiver feels the tug of competing obligations. Like some 28 percent of caregivers in America, I'm one of the so-called sandwich generation.[1] Although the term was coined to indicate a caregiver for both young children and elderly parents, its reach has expanded to include those like me, caring for both children and a spouse (am I an open-face sandwich?), and indeed any caregiver with multiple charges of different ages. In *Why We Can't Sleep*, Ada Calhoun offers the term "the caregiving rack" for this phenomenon, nicely evoking the image of being stretched thin.[2] Nonwhite caregivers, it's important to note, are significantly more likely to have children or grandchildren living with them: whereas 24 percent of white caregivers have kids in the home, that figure is 34 percent for both Black and Asian American caregivers and 38 percent in the Latinx caregiving community.[3]

When I was coordinating all aspects of life for both my husband and my children, I felt like I was playing emotional and logistical Twister. The goals I was reaching for, though, weren't big blue or yellow dots. Instead the commands would have been: Get the kids to school without yelling at them! Take Brad to a doctor's appointment and act calm in front of the doctors! Make sure there's milk in the fridge and clean clothes for tomorrow! Rearrange the kids' counseling appointments, which are at the same office, so they overlap instead of requiring separate trips! Any one of those tasks is nothing much by itself, but put all together they stretched me to the max.

A LACK OF REASONABLE OPTIONS

The ways these various pulls manifest are as complex as family structures themselves. Sandwiched caregiving can look any number of different ways. The archetypal version might be a middle-aged woman caring for both aging parents and her young children. As we saw in chapter 5, the average caregiver is a forty-nine-year-old woman—and these days many forty-nine-year-olds have younger kids at home. In the article "Caught in the Middle: Caring for Your Kids and Your Aging Parents," Laura

Richards provides a memorable portrait of (and tips for surviving) the sandwiched life: "I was heavily pregnant with my fourth and final child when my very fit seventy-one-year-old father, who frequently ran road races, had a devastating stroke," she writes. She suggests having important conversations about medical decisions with parents before they're needed and preventing burnout by setting boundaries for getting through such a high-need situation.[4]

Lorene Cary's recent memoir *Ladysitting* offers a poignant self-portrait of sandwiched caregiving.[5] At the book's outset Cary's beloved Nana, a centenarian, still lives in her own home in the Philadelphia suburbs. Cary has a teenage daughter at home and another college-aged daughter nearby; she runs an arts nonprofit and lives in Philadelphia, half an hour's drive from Nana's house. Going back and forth to check up on her takes a toll, and when Nana contracts a bladder infection she can no longer live independently. Cary and her family have space to take her in, thanks to her husband Bob's work as a pastor: they live in a large rectory. But it is a strain to accommodate the high needs of an extremely particular woman who requires near-constant care. Intergenerational conflict adds to the challenge: Cary's grandmother does not speak to Cary's father (her son), so caregiving must skip a generation. Cary interweaves her story of caregiving with her Black family history—her grandmother comes from an old free Black family from North Carolina—and the particular, difficult legacies of this personal history and trauma.

The book's opening juxtaposes Cary's warm childhood memories of her grandparents' house with a clear-eyed look at Nana's now-failing health. Cary loves her grandmother deeply and is committed to caring for her, to giving her the good death that her dignity and age deserve. Yet doing so becomes increasingly difficult. Cary feels like her divided attentions are shortchanging everyone, herself included. Nana wants full-time devotion, an endless need that Cary links to Nana's losing her mother at the age of six. To satisfy Nana's demands, Cary's daughters must pitch in: the older by living alone in Nana's crumbling suburban house, which Nana refuses to sell, the younger by "ladysitting" her great-grandmother while Cary is at work. Cary writes movingly about how she is missing time with her teen daughter, at one point wishing simply to take a couple of hours to watch a movie together. *Ladysitting* conveys beautifully the impact of eldercare not just on the caregiver but on an entire family system.

I've seen the theme pop up, too, in popular fiction like Allison Pearson's *How Hard Can It Be?*, a sequel to her hit *I Don't Know How She Does It*, a British comedy of manners about the pressures of being a working mother. *I Don't Know How She Does It* struck a chord when it came out in 2002, with its opening scene of the sleep-deprived heroine, Kate Reddy, gently distressing store-bought pies so they would look homemade for the school bake sale.

In the 2015 sequel, Kate is forty-nine (there's that average-caregiver age again) and struggling to hold it all together (troubled teen kids, house renovations, a husband changing careers) when her elderly mother has a fall. Kate must rush to her side for the immediate crisis and then try to manage nursing help from afar. On top of this she must also assist with the needs of her in-laws. The strain of long-distance caregiving manifests in Kate's worries about her mother's care: "Please observe how strenuously nice I am to the nurse! My face aches from using every reserve of charm I possess. . . . I need her to like me because I am about to leave my mother in her hands, and I fear that, if I annoy her for some reason . . . she could take it out on Mum."[6] Kate's frantic inner state comes across as she vents to a man who tells her she should take a break: "I worry all the time about my children, my daughter especially; I worry about my mum, my sister, my husband's parents, my best friend who's basically a functioning alcoholic, my dog, my work, my health . . . it's all too much. I can't break free, I just can't."[7] Her own health—anything to do with her personally—is down at the bottom, two notches below her dog.

Like all caregiving, sandwiched caregiving is gendered. As Darcy Lockman notes in *All the Rage*, studies show that adult daughters are more likely than their brothers to help aging parents with emotionally and physically demanding tasks such as bathing and feeding. These tasks are more likely to interrupt the caregivers' lives, whereas men tend to perform flexible, occasional services like grocery shopping and yard work: "When it comes to setting their personal priorities aside, be it for their children or their parents, women are the generous sex," Lockman writes.[8]

Any sandwiched caregiver will likely feel caught between their two responsibilities—or maybe overstretched. I never could decide which metaphor was more fitting: the feeling of being pressed, like ham in a panini, or of being stretched thin, like taffy. Multigenerational and multidirectional caring—for instance, caring for friends or neighbors in addition to family members—comes with unique challenges.

I have friends, a couple, who had a newborn within days of the non-childbearing parent's emergency surgery for cancer, which was followed by chemotherapy. The postpartum parent cared for her spouse, for their older child, and for their newborn all at once. I remember exchanging emails with her when I was facing Brad's stem cell transplant, with its long hospitalization. How, I asked her, had she gotten through it? I never forgot her answer: a lack of any other reasonable options. There was no choice but to do all the necessary things to keep everyone moving forward. I thought about that answer all the time when I got the kids ready for school or decided not to drive to the airport to run away, and it was strangely comforting. There was no reasonable option but to keep going. People needed me to—people I love. And so I did.

Another old friend of mine, more recently, has faced a top-heavy sort of sandwich (a pot pie?). She has one daughter—about the same age as my daughter Lucy—and a plethora of older relatives who need help, and the whole family was deeply affected by the devastating Camp Fire of 2018. The pressure of it all sounds unimaginably intense.

I often wonder at how my imagination fails when I look at the caregiving challenges of others. I know they had the same reaction to me when I was juggling Brad's intense care needs and parenthood, and I remember my own feelings going through it. But because every situation is unique, my memories don't always translate into understanding how a friend is getting through their own caregiving situation. Nor, in truth, does it help me know how to help them. As long as the US model of the solo family caregiver persists, there aren't many ways to truly relieve the pressure on sandwiched caregivers. Every situation looks different and impossible from the outside. From the inside, you muddle through.

The expectations around who has what sociologists would call a "status obligation" to provide care differ widely among cultures, producing different care and sandwiching scenarios. Sometimes cultural norms aim to sidestep sandwiching altogether: for instance, Laura Esquivel's novel *Like Water for Chocolate* depicts a traditional Mexican expectation that a youngest daughter will remain unmarried and childless so she can care for her parents in old age—an expectation driving the plot. In many Asian cultures, elders have high status,[9] with adult children—and particularly daughters-in-law—expected to provide care. Ai-jen Poo notes: "China and other East Asian countries . . . strongly believe that with age comes elevated status, and the corresponding responsibility of younger family members to care for their elders and ancestors."[10] The recent movie *The Farewell* is a moving look at caregiving in China, particularly how assumptions around caring for the elderly are different from those in the United States. In the film a family refuses to tell its matriarch she has been diagnosed with terminal cancer, much to the bafflement of the Chinese American granddaughter, played by Awkwafina. Instead, the family organizes a fake wedding to enable everyone to say their goodbyes while hiding the diagnosis from the patient. In the US, it would be unthinkable not to disclose such a critical piece of medical information; in China, as depicted in the movie (based on real events in director Lulu Wang's family), family decisions are paramount—but the family shares a duty to care for its elder.

In the African American community, multiple caring obligations have historically been common. In the antebellum era one's personally chosen, family-oriented care often coexisted with—and was sadly compromised by—the care that enslaved Black women were forced to provide to nonrelatives. In our current era Black and other nonwhite women often work as domestic care workers, with long hours and low pay making it harder to care for their own family. A paradigmatic example of this bind comes from immigrant women working as caregivers or nannies to support family in their home country. Such workers cannot personally care for their own families, at great emotional cost to all concerned—yet they are sandwiched caregivers nonetheless, thanks to economic pressures.

The expense of providing for children at home is an obvious further strain for sandwiched caregivers. Those who are both caregiving and caring for children are doubly likely to miss work, curtail their work hours, or step out of the workforce altogether. Added to that, the AARP Public Policy Institute and National Alliance for Caregiving report, *Caregiving in the US*, reveals that two demographic groups most likely to be sandwiched—Black and Latinx caregivers—have significantly lower median incomes than white or Asian American caregivers.[11]

Although broad cultural values shape the ways individual families provide care, there are enormous individual variations based on circumstance, choice, and interpersonal dynamics. These choices can be fraught, as in Indian Canadian writer Rohinton Mistry's sprawling, moving novel

Family Matters. In it, a Parsi family in Bombay is caring for the patriarch, Nariman, who has Parkinson's disease. When Nariman falls and breaks his leg, the family erupts in conflict. Nariman's stepdaughter, who has been caring for him but resents him, pushes her younger, less well-off half-sister Roxana to take him in. Roxana is kinder and more loving than her sibling—but she and her husband have two children and live in a cramped apartment. Her sons become closer to their grandfather but financial and marital strains erupt: in one scene summing up the tension, Roxana's son Jehangir overhears his father yelling at his mother: "'I didn't marry you for the honour and privilege of nursing your father.'"[12] It's telling that at the center of a book called *Family Matters* is a question of who will care for an elder: caring for each other is the essence of family.

In other representations the valences of family caregiving can differ from expectations. Alice Walker's *The Color Purple* turns on a story of enforced sandwiched caregiving, which radically restructures the Black family at the novel's center—and becomes a force of liberation for the main character. Set in the Jim Crow South, the novel follows Celie, who is molested as a child and married to an abusive husband. Celie is starved for human connection, having been separated from her beloved sister Nettie. The downtrodden, often exploited Celie has long been tending her husband's children as their stepmother. She then must care for her husband's ailing mistress, the glamorous (and scandalous) blues singer Shug Avery, whom her husband brings home to recover from an unspecified illness. Shug is at first "hateful"—"sick as she is, if a snake cross her path, she kill it"[13]—and resistant to care, but through tending to her, Celie finds love.

One scene of Celie caring for Shug, combing her hair, might be the tenderest portrait of caregiving I've ever read: "I work on her like she a doll or like she Olivia—or like she mama. I comb and pat, comb and pat. First she say, hurry up and git finish. Then she melt down a little and lean back gainst my knees. That feel just right, she say. That feel like mama used to do. Or maybe not mama. Maybe grandma."[14] The Olivia mentioned here is Celie's lost daughter, born when her stepfather raped Celie as a child and later given away by the same stepfather. This scene, to me, highlights the common pleasures and human side between caregiving for the ill and for a child. For Celie connection like this has been rare, and she falls deeply in love with Shug, who in turn encourages her to find her own worth.

Celie also has other caring obligations: since childhood she has been forced to tend to children (first her siblings, then her stepchildren), and she cares for her stepson Harpo's wife, Sofia, after a white mob has beaten her nearly to death. Sofia, in jail, has no access to medical care and Celie's description of her injuries is harrowing: "When I see Sofia I don't know why she still alive. They crack her skull, they crack her ribs. They tear her nose loose on one side. They blind her. In one eye. She swole from head to foot. Her tongue the size of my arm, it stick out tween her teef like a piece of rubber." The only tools Celie has to nurse her in the jail cell are "witch hazel and alcohol" and water to wash, brought by the "colored 'tendant."[15] Sofia's crime was to say she didn't want to be a white woman's maid.

The care that Celie gives Sofia in jail illustrates the care networks that marginalized communities must often form. Care networks of this type date to when Black Americans were enslaved: mothers or other family members, forced to work, could not necessarily care for their own kin—and slave owners offered no access to doctors—so healthcare became communal. Such a model of a marginalized community coming together to care for its own is analogous to the type of collective caregiving that has emerged under very different conditions for LGBTQ communities in recent decades (discussed in chapter 5).

Briallen Hopper's account of co-caregiving with a friend group is clear about the challenges that her sandwiched co-caregivers face: "Among the care team, I was exceptional and lucky in that for years Ash's illness was my only substantial caregiving responsibility, and my sole source of mortal grief and dread."[16] Other friends on the team cared for and lost in-laws, had babies, and in one case worked full-time as a chaplain at a trauma center. Caregivers who have emotionally taxing jobs may be even more at risk of care burnout.

Although such networks have been built out of necessity, I wonder if the idea of distributing the responsibility of care can help to ease the stress of sandwiched caregiving.

THE EVERYDAY JUGGLE

For me the demands of caregiving with kids have faded considerably since the time Brad seemed to be dying but they can still flare up. During the time I was working on this chapter, Brad had cataract surgery. It was June

2019, the beginning of summer vacation for our daughters. Cataract surgery, a relatively minor outpatient procedure, is the most commonly performed surgery in the developed world.[17] (Then again, everyone who gets it gets it twice.) For Brad, in the wake of his cancer treatment, however, nothing is really minor. He gets terribly anxious about medical procedures, remembering all the trauma he's already endured. Anesthetic hits him hard, and with his suppressed immune system, infections are always a worry.

In the years since his cancer diagnosis, we've come a long way in terms of reducing the care he needs and the work it places on me, but on the day of the cataract surgery it felt like we were right back at square one. He had to be dropped off at the same-day surgery center, and I needed to be on standby for picking him up. Our younger daughter, then nine, was home and bored. Our older daughter, shortly to turn fourteen, had gone away to summer camp with a friend and was due back in Sacramento sometime around when the surgery was scheduled to finish. It was unclear when I would need to pick her up.

Brad had slept poorly and was in a tense, foul mood in the morning when it was time to go to the surgery center. I mixed up the time, thinking he needed to get dropped off at 9:30 when it was really 9:15. We raced over, a little late, after I took a shower, which got delayed because Lucy wanted me to make her breakfast and my gym session ran a little long. In between I was texting my mother-in-law to share the timing of the surgery. Lucy decided she desperately wanted to bake a chocolate cake, and though I initially said no, I eventually caved. I regretted it when every single instruction in the recipe caused her to call out "MOM?" for help and clarification.

At 11:30, a nurse at the surgery center called: Brad was out of surgery and I should come get him. At exactly the same moment Lucy summoned me, frantic, to take the cake out of the oven. I still wasn't sure when Nora was getting back from the summer camp but I'd been told to expect to pick her up any minute, so I texted the other mom, my friend Amy. No response. I knew Amy had to return to work soon after getting back to town, so I worried I was sticking her with my kid—but I had to go get Brad. As I was getting into my car to head to the surgery center the nurse called again, now huffy, to say that Brad was ready for pickup. Just as I pulled into the surgery center Nora texted to say she was back and waiting to be picked up. Nothing I could do about that. (In the end, Amy dropped her off at home.)

When I got to Brad's recovery bedside he was extremely groggy and in no condition to go anywhere: his IV was still in place, a hospital gown still on, and the nurses busy with other patients. An hour later we were back on our way home, where—ravenous by then—I ate the remnants of Lucy's microwaved ravioli for lunch.

I fixed Brad some Jell-O, explained his eyedrop regimen and told him he was supposed to keep an eye shield on until the next morning, helped with the first round of eye drops, kicked Lucy off the computer where she was watching God knew what on YouTube, and then headed out to pick up a birthday present for Nora and some dinner. Nobody ended up liking the takeout food much, everyone was tired, and by evening I felt frustrated and angry with Brad, who I suddenly noticed wasn't wearing the eye shield. He didn't like the tape on his face; he planned to wear sunglasses to sleep instead. I was worried about the potential for infection; the glasses had been floating around in his none-too-clean backpack. A friend had told me about how her mom's cataract surgery had gone awry when she contracted a staph infection—the eye turned black and she lost vision permanently. I was trying mightily to keep that horror story to myself and not share it with Brad, whose anxiety didn't need feeding. But I wanted him to follow the doctor's instructions, which he hadn't heard in his postsurgery anesthetic haze.

The disagreement turned bitter: I felt like the work and care I'd lavished on him was being wasted, he felt like I was infantilizing him, and we started yelling. Lucy came downstairs crying to tell me not to yell at Daddy. Soon all of us were crying, but I couldn't let the stupid eye-patch quarrel go. The whole situation had, for me, triggered all of the anger and frustration of the past few years and I couldn't rein it in. I felt badly sandwiched, so pressed by what I saw as Brad's health needs that I couldn't pull back to attend to my kids' emotional needs.

What I had most wanted to do on that day of competing family demands was sit down and work on this book. The day before I'd had a great writing day and I wanted to keep the momentum going, but naturally I barely had so much as a chance to keep up with email. Stop, start, stop, start: the familiar rhythm of work during the years of intense mothering, compounded by caregiving. I wrote this paragraph while Lucy was at a friend's house and Brad was resting on the couch the day after the cataract surgery.

That whole logistical hassle was far from the most serious one of Brad's treatment but it felt like acute irony to be squished between the competing demands of my husband's medical needs and our kids while writing this chapter. It brought up sharp memories of caring for everyone and everything during a more fragile time.

When Brad's illness became acute I canceled the girls' activities right and left: piano and gymnastics were early casualties. Some shows, however, had to go on, like the production of *Annie* in which Nora had been cast when Brad was first hospitalized. The hardest choices were the emotional tugs. We had to rehome Lucy's beloved but destructive cat Charley when it became clear Brad needed a transplant; for reasons of immune suppression we couldn't have a pet in the home for a full year during his recovery.

I had briefly faced a more classic caregiving sandwich several years before, when my mother was in the last months of her life before her death by suicide. She became manic and then deeply depressed around the time Lucy was born. She had been helping me by caring for our older daughter but now she herself needed care. She, in her turn, had recently emerged from the strain of caring for my grandfather, who had had Parkinson's—a challenge that I think contributed to her growing instability.

One day she called me, crying, from her therapist's office. She had told him of her suicidal urges and he wouldn't let her go home without assurance someone would be with her. I stayed with her for a day, found companionship for her, and looked for a better psychiatrist. I did all of this in the fog of someone whose infant was waking up five or six times a night. Sadly, my experience caring for my mother was brief—her suicide occurred a month later. That short experience, however, gave me a vivid insight into the demands of caring for a truly dependent elder as well as small children.

Thinking about my experience with my mother prompted me to reflect on the difficult, varying demands of providing different types of care for different types of illness. Caregiving for mental illness is rarely acknowledged, extraordinarily emotionally taxing, and often surrounded by feelings of shame. And it's even less well supported than other types of caregiving, as Mira T. Lee depicts in her novel *Everything Here Is Beautiful.* The novel, told from multiple points of view, follows the charismatic but unstable character Lucia Bok through her romantic relationships, young motherhood, and painful breakdowns. An especially poignant moment comes when Lucia's husband, Manny, is trying to help her, but she is refusing her medications. Manny has promised himself he'll try to save Lucia, mainly for their daughter's sake: "He had kept the promise a long, long time. He had stuck by Lucia. This was love, or this was duty, he could no longer tell the difference."[18]

As Manny's plight shows, the challenges for both patients and caregivers can be exacerbated if the patient is combative, delusional, or estranged from close family. My mother, for instance, was often hostile or angry with me, and we were briefly estranged during Lucy's infancy. My kids were too young then to understand the emotional strain of my mom's mental illness. That wasn't the case during Brad's cancer treatment, though I think we still haven't fully grappled with its effects on them. Meeting their emotional need for security was a constant challenge. I sometimes drained myself trying to compensate for the things Brad used to do with them: tossing Lucy up in the air over and over during long summer days at the neighborhood pool, catching for her as she practiced softball pitching, helping dig little ditches so they could run water in from the creek at the cabin. I wanted to soften the blow of their functionally missing dad as much as I could.

LEAVING GEORGE DONNER

As I confronted the difficult choices Brad's treatment foisted on our family, I thought of a strange parallel: the tragic fate of the infamous Donner Party, the emigrants who left Springfield, Illinois, in 1846 to try to reach Sutter's Fort in what is now Sacramento, where I live. The Donner Party took an unproven and disastrous shortcut on the trail and failed to make their way out of the Sierra Nevada mountains before an early snowfall trapped them. To survive (which many of them ultimately did not), the Donners and the other families with them ate shoe leather and grass and eventually one another. Most people tend to focus on the cannibalism when they think about the Donner Party, which is understandable; it's sensational, horrifying. But for me, of all of the Donner Party's mysteries, the one that haunts me most is the fate of Tamsen Donner, the wife of George Donner, coleader of the group with James Reed. In early 1847 a small group of the strongest survivors made their way on foot to the valley below (several dying en route) and rescuers from Sutter's Fort set out to try to guide some remaining survivors to the safety of the valley. George Donner was dying, far too weak to make the trek, and so Tamsen and their children stayed behind with him. When a second rescue party arrived in early March, Tamsen sent her daughters—Frances, Georgia, and Eliza, ages six, four, and three—with the rescuers and stayed with her dying husband, a choice amounting to suicide. Indeed, neither survived; the fourth rescue expedition in April found George Donner dead in his bed and no trace of Tamsen.

What was Tamsen Donner thinking? There were no relatives waiting for the little girls in Alta California, then contested territory in the Mexican-American War. Maybe she had an outsized faith in her own ability to get out. Maybe she was so addled by hopeless isolation that she didn't care anymore. There's no way to know. But I know this: I would not make that choice.

The pressures of sandwiched caregiving, and how easily it can crush the caregiver, are starkly illuminated by Tamsen's choice. It also underscores the gulf between attitudes to marriage then and now. Then, a woman's place was by her husband's side, even unto death: she was wife first, mother second, person last of all. Today, the order is reversed. People of my generation are individuals before they are spouses. I have given up many things I love during my husband's illness (career, travel, sex) but I've always protected the essential parts of my self. Self-erasure is no longer required of women who love.

When Brad was already sick, but not yet diagnosed, in 2015, we both accompanied our elder daughter on a field trip that was the highlight of fourth grade: a living-history overnight at Sutter's Fort. Meant to re-create conditions in the days of 1847, the field trip included each kid picking a character of someone at the fort in those days. Everyone dressed in pioneer-style clothes; I ordered dresses off of Etsy and we took a picture of all of us, unsmiling like in a daguerreotype, Brad thinner than usual because of what we didn't yet know was cancer.

Sutter's Fort was the outpost that the Donners and company were trying to reach. Some of them, including those young Donner girls, did; many didn't. Our daughter chose the persona of Margaret Reed, the wife of George Donner's coleader James Reed. None of the Reeds starved. Margaret Reed saved sugar for a Christmas treat and husbanded (the word should really be wived) the food carefully, keeping it hidden from many of the others in the party. (I thought of Reed when, hunkering down for a long period of isolation during the coronavirus crisis, I hid a box of my daughters' favorite chocolate-covered marshmallows at the back of the pantry cupboard.) She protected her children, fiercely. (The Reed children later would claim theirs was the only family that didn't eat human flesh.) Tamsen Donner was less provident than Margaret Reed and saved less food.

I became fascinated with the insight into Tamsen Donner as both a real and a fictionalized character in Gabrielle Burton's novel *Impatient with Desire*, which interleaves Tamsen's imagined journal with passages from her real letters. Burton also wrote a memoir, *Searching for Tamsen Donner*, about her obsession with the Donner matriarch, whom she takes as an object lesson. "Without my intention or even my notice," Burton writes in *Searching*, "Tamsen Donner became entwined, warp and woof, with my struggle to become a . . . A what? Not a mother who wrote; that sounds like a hobby or a sideline. Not a writer who mothered; that also sounds part-time. My husband wasn't a professor who fathered or a father who taught; he just was both. That's what I struggled for, just to be both: a writer and a mother, and vice versa, giving equal weight to both, as men do."[19] Burton, a generation older than I, writes about the 1970s as the time she struggled with this dilemma. I've struggled with this tension between children and career as well, but until I began caregiving, I—naively, as I discussed in chapter 1—never really thought of my married status as a fundamental part of my identity: marriage hadn't felt like it changed who I was on a deep level the way that motherhood, say, had. But the demands of caring for Brad clarified the extent to which my marriage shaped my choices and how it could clash deeply with other choices I might make for personal or professional fulfillment.

Tamsen Donner struggled not with the tension between motherhood and professional fulfillment, but with the conflict between her roles as a mother and as a wife. She prioritized her role as wife. In both Burton's fictional account and in real life, staying behind as Tamsen did was a suicide mission (though we know that she did try to cross the mountains alone after George's death). I can't understand choosing a dying man, and death for myself, over my young children. I can't imagine my husband wanting me to. Is this a failure of love or imagination, a sign I haven't cleaved to my husband enough?

As my husband grew sicker and his treatment longer, I leaned more and more toward choosing the girls: pulling them from aftercare to be with them in the evenings instead of staying with him at the hospital, taking them on trips though he was not healthy enough to join, chaperoning a field trip instead of attending an appointment with the oncologist. I have withdrawn, bit by bit, from the bond with my husband and focused, bit by bit, more on our daughters and myself.

The question of whom to choose became starker during Brad's treatment for the Epstein-Barr cancer. He was getting infusions of a drug called Rituxan,[20] which seemed to be reducing the cancer load—but Dr. T did not think it would provide a long-term cure. A clinical trial he found, however, did offer hope for such a cure. The catch? It was in New York, and Brad would have to live there for several weeks, for most of December. Treatment would be paid for; transportation, lodging, and assistance for navigating an unfamiliar city at a time when he was visually impaired would not. His parents, always generous, offered to help. The question was whether they or I would go with him to New York.

The choice was mine and I chose to stay home. I wasn't giving up on my husband but I was preparing for the worst with our girls in mind. They had already experienced their father's illness as an abandonment, however unintentional; they would have experienced my going to New York for the clinical trial, at Christmas, the same way. Less nobly, I was also tired of cancer dominating our lives, and a few weeks at home with the girls sounded almost like a break.

And so, guilt mixed with relief, I sent my ill, weak, visually impaired husband alone on a plane to New York, flying over the spot where the Donners had huddled miserably, in a rough snow shanty cobbled together from fir branches and the canvas wagon top, 170 years before. He lay not in a jolting wagon but in JetBlue's first-class service, where passengers have a personal adjustable, fully reclining chair for their comfort. He said it was great.

It seemed to me like a huge step to put him on that plane. His parents were there to meet him on the other end. We all had new hope he might survive—which in the end he did. In Sacramento I felt like I was in the wilderness still, as numb as the Donners' extremities must have been. But while he was gone I had a bit of freedom. I put away the medications cluttering our dining room. I took the girls off to school every morning and settled in for six hours of time to myself. I wrote. I took baths. I spent one whole day in a bathrobe watching movies and felt guilty. But I was myself. I was a better, more patient mother, a happier person. The girls and I fell into an easy rhythm, into which I doled out surprise treats: I took them to see *The Nutcracker*, we went out for rich hot chocolate at our favorite confectioner (a few blocks from Sutter's Fort), we watched *The Great British Bake Off* during dinner. I felt both uncomfortable about and reassured by the sneaking feeling this interlude was like practice in case we had to become a family of three.

That brief respite showed me clearly how corrosive the strain of caregiving had been. What are the bounds of marriage and selfhood? I thought about Paul Simon's song "Hearts and Bones," about his stormy relationship with Carrie Fisher. My mother played that song endlessly after my father left her, as she cried. During the times of greatest strain while Brad was at his sickest, when I thought often about leaving him, I remembered that our hearts and our bones are twirled together, as the song says—in our case, in our children—and that bond will never come undone. If I left, I wondered, would it damage the girls more than if I stayed, unhappy, expending my life on Brad's suffering?

So far our girls and I haven't needed the practice we got being on our own. The Rituxan knocked back that Epstein-Barr cancer, and the clinical trial finished the job. It hasn't come back, and our anguish at Dr. T's pronouncement of Brad having a year or less to live has evaporated—or rather, has been filed away in those places where our shared and different traumas from Brad's illness live, deep within us. We are still a family of four, and both of my husband's cancers are in remission, a phrase to which I always add a superstitious "for now." He still has chronic graft-versus-host disease; he has had to retire from his career because of the consequent disability; and his life span is almost certainly shortened. We don't know if he will live long enough to see the girls' graduations or weddings or whatever milestones may lie ahead. For that matter, we don't know if I will; there are no guarantees.

A few months after Brad came home from New York, I got a stomach bug. When I did, Brad was able to walk to the store and buy me ginger ale and saltines. It felt like the beginning of hope and a beginning of healing for us both, as well as for the kids.

All caregiving relationships may bring a crossroads where the needs of the ill person become so extreme that there's no room for self. In such cases I believe it's courageous to find a balance affording the caregiver some respite. Lorene Cary describes such a crossroads in *Ladysitting*. Cary has promised to care for Nana at home rather than moving her into a facility but the strain mounts when, toward the end of the year, Nana has become paranoid and insists on firing a trusted paid caregiver. She isn't sleeping and neither is Cary, who senses that she's reached the end of her rope—but she comes to the realization with a heavy load of familial obligation underlying it: "I needed sleep to knit up the ragged ends of rage, of not getting my own, of never being enough to satisfy her, as I felt I hadn't satisfied my parents, and ancestors who demanded redemption through their offspring."[21] Cary, overwhelmed and overstretched, breaks the promise she has made, calling a family respite care program at a local hospital even though she fears Nana will hate her for it: "Push had come to shove, and I'd chosen me and mine over her. This is what Nana had been telling me I'd do. For years."[22] But in a surprising, kind irony, Nana's days at the respite care center slide into hospice care and the peaceful, relatively comfortable death her granddaughter sought for her. Nana dies with Cary and her younger daughter next to her, a bittersweet resolution to this multigenerational caregiving story.

This kind of generational harmony is something that newer models of caregiving seek. I was struck in reading Ai-jen Poo's *The Age of Dignity* by Poo's call for innovative cross-generational models of care. My own challenges with caring for Brad and our children were tremendously eased by the presence of his parents throughout the most acute phases of his illness; we were fortunate that my in-laws were robustly healthy in their seventies. But, as Poo points out, even frail elders can still participate in looking after their grandchildren, and grandchildren (teens especially) can help elders whose care needs don't yet extend to nursing tasks or heavy assistance.[23] What some caregiving advocates call a "care village" can apply this model of cross-generational community care more broadly to kids and elders who are not related but may have complementary needs.

BURNED SANDWICH

Such a sea change, however, seems far away in the current climate. Because there is so little support of this kind, sandwiched caregivers and others with multiple care responsibilities may be especially vulnerable to burnout. In a 2009 study, Rose Rubin and Shelley I. White-Means found lower overall quality of life among sandwiched caregivers of elderly parents, in comparison to those caregivers without children at home.[24] Interestingly, they found that for sandwiched caregivers, employment provided some relief of stress, suggesting breaks from high-demand caregiving duties as well as an independent sense of self and purpose are critical to caregiver well-being. The question is how to get those breaks and find time to foster that purpose.

Much is made in the caregiving literature of the importance of self-care, which has unfortunately been translated in the popular consciousness as self-indulgence—a conception spurred on by misogynist associations and cynical marketing. But bubble baths and mani-pedis, while pleasant, aren't a full picture of self-care, which Audre Lorde called "an act of political warfare."[25] *Bitch* editor Evette Dionne, writing in *Ravishly*, discusses how self-care continues to be a radical act for Black women. "Self-care is a radical feminist act for Black women because we've spent generations in servitude to others. In fact, Black women have often been considered properties of our communities," Dionne writes. "We're conditioned to believe that we're obligated to nurture others at our own expense."[26] Shanesha Brooks-Tatum, writing on Feminist Wire, links this idea to the history of Black women in slavery: "It's subversive to take care of ourselves because for centuries black women worldwide have been taking care of others, from the children of slave masters to those of business executives, and often serving today as primary caregivers for the elderly as home health workers and nursing home employees."[27]

The extreme strain that caregiving, both paid and unpaid, places on Black women and other women of color is something that no amount of self-care can fully alleviate. But, I would argue, for women who must care for others it does become radical to place at least equal value on caring for themselves. Although white and more privileged caregivers like me must not appropriate the language of activism or make the mistake of imagining getting a massage is a radical thing to do, perhaps we can take the lesson that carving out space for both individual self-preservation and collective action will help women in any caring role. As we've already seen, caregiver burnout is real. And its effects can be surprisingly long-lasting—for both the care recipient and the stressed or even traumatized caregiver.

EIGHT

SOMETHING IS NOT RIGHT

Post-Caregiving Stress

Home from New York and in remission, Brad began a new life of recovering from the trauma of cancer and coping with his ongoing chronic illness. His disability retirement went into effect in February 2017 and he became a full-time patient instead, with frequent treatments, blood tests, and doctor visits. Although he wasn't acutely ill we had to be constantly vigilant for flares of GvHD or signs of infection. Even a low fever could land him in the hospital; infections were a constant worry, and obsessive handwashing and sanitizing were the rule in our house long before the coronavirus made them de rigueur. His impaired vision continued to be a challenge; although his scarred eyes had improved a bit, he would need corneal transplants to recover more of his sight.

It was hard to get back to a state I could think of as normal when so many medical dangers still lurked for him. We had already seen so many surprises and reversals in his treatment that I'd come to doubt any medical professional who reassured us. Brad never, it seemed, could get the normal, average, expected ailment. He always had something rare, the thing that surprised the doctors and brought the specialists to his hospital room saying they'd never seen this before. I was well trained in hypervigilance.

One day, about a year after he came home from New York, Brad started to cough and his energy level dropped hard. It turned out to be pneumonia—one of the many conditions requiring automatic hospitalization for a stem cell transplant survivor. It amazed me at the time how quickly I snapped into what I think of as hospital mode. It all felt so familiar, so well-oiled, so natural: Call the hospital. Pressure them to get a room open. Pack a bag. Rearrange everyone's schedule. Reassure the kids. Take extra hospital socks. Let our families know what's going on. The patterns we developed at the height of his illness will always be with us. Even though the demands of my husband's illness are nowhere near as severe as they used to be, knowing that any day he could get pneumonia, or have a flare-up, or have an anxiety-producing scan ordered, can feel like a lot. The resources for processing all of that and for living with uncertainty—never my strongest suit—don't feel quite adequate to the strain. I'm not sure what would help; maybe all of life is strain and we have to press on as best we can.

That hospital stay for pneumonia lasted only three days. Everything went smoothly. Unlike with Brad's first emergency three years before, there were no hideous surprises like a collapsed lung, and it didn't start out with the terrifying shock of him suddenly coughing up blood. But that first hospitalization is what set in motion our patterns around his illness. I was the driver, reassuring him, tamping down my own panic so that I could be Good in a Crisis. I asked questions, pushed staff for answers, kept going, was reassuring. When such emergencies come up again I almost feel like I'm taking up arms, even if sometimes all I've got is lipstick and a fully charged phone.

As you know I hate the military metaphors that frame cancer as a battle, but one thing that combat and severe illness do have in common is that both produce trauma. There's starting to be more recognition that survivors of severe illness can exhibit post-traumatic stress disorder (PTSD), a condition that is most often linked to war veterans but in fact occurs much more widely, and for more varied reasons.[1] I by no means claim that diagnosis for all caregivers but I do think there can be trauma involved for families as well as patients. Whatever the clinical terminology, a prolonged caregiving experience can have significant reverberations in people's lives, even after the intense responsibilities of caregiving fade. The economic penalties on caregivers discussed in chapter 6, for instance, persist long after the bills have been paid, including the reduction of Social Security or retirement income because of fewer working hours accrued. Social aftereffects can stem from the isolation of caregiving, with relationships weakened temporarily or permanently. Linked to this social and relationship damage—but for me deeper and perhaps even more persistent—are the emotional effects of intense caregiving. These can include hypervigilance, ongoing anger or irritation, and depression or despair. I felt and sometimes still feel like I'd lost my self in the care of others, and a recovery from that feeling—especially in the midst of my husband's ongoing chronic illness—has been elusive.

POST-TRAUMATIC STRESS: WHAT IT IS, WHAT IT ISN'T

All of these symptoms, taken together, sound a bit like the commonly accepted definition of PTSD. The US Department of Veterans Affairs does significant outreach about PTSD and the overview on its website provides an accessible introduction to the scope of the disorder: "PTSD is a mental health problem that some people develop after experiencing or witnessing a life-threatening event, like combat, a natural disaster, a car accident, or sexual assault. It's normal to have upsetting memories, feel on edge, or have trouble sleeping after this type of event. If symptoms last more than a few months, it may be PTSD."[2] The diagnostic criteria for PTSD were broadened in 2013 within the fifth edition of the American Psychiatric Association's *Diagnostic and Statistical Manual* (*DSM-5*), which also placed the condition within a newly created category of trauma- and stressor-related disorders. Previously, PTSD had been classified as an anxiety disorder. That shift, as the APA notes, acknowledges that the condition is "increasingly at the center of public as well as professional discussion."[3] The triggering event for PTSD may have nothing to do with military service: one in three cancer survivors, for instance, shows at least one PTSD symptom cluster.[4]

Unfortunately PTSD has become a term often tossed off casually to indicate unpleasant reminders: a quick Twitter search yields joking references to PTSD from toxic relationships, the *Jurassic Park* theme song, and physics class. I know I've used the term in the same kind of minimizing way in the past. The same search, however, which I ran on the anniversary of Hurricane Katrina, also turned up many serious examples related to that disaster, and several online exchanges with PTSD sufferers telling those who use the term flippantly to knock it off.

Where does this leave those who experience caregiving as a kind of secondhand trauma? Although the diagnostic standards for PTSD have wider application than they once did, they remain stringent: there are eight categories of criteria—starting with type of stressor, which can include witnessing trauma—and all must be met for diagnosis. The criteria also include intrusive symptoms such as flashbacks, avoidance of trauma reminders, feelings of isolation, overly negative thoughts, reactivity (such as hypervigilance or irritation), and duration of symptoms for more than a month.[5]

Often, what many caregivers suffer from is not PTSD but rather post-traumatic stress (PTS): not a disorder, but an ongoing reaction to strain. PTS can overlap with the symptoms of PTSD but usually improves on its own, without treatment.[6] However, PTS can be a precursor to the development of full-blown PTSD. A 2005 study of 459 intensive-care patients found significant post-traumatic stress symptoms in a third of family caregivers interviewed. It can be difficult to obtain a diagnosis of any kind of syndrome after caregiving—not just because the situation doesn't fit traditional models of trauma, but also because caregivers are less likely to seek out healthcare.

For some, the very experience of diagnosis can evoke difficult feelings, as British writer Ella Risbridger (whose other work on caregiving is discussed in chapter 2) outlined in her 2020 newsletter *You Get in Love and Then You Die*: "Getting a diagnosis with my particular flavour of PTSD was near impossible: I am phobic about doctors, about hospitals, about tests, about results, about anything—in short—even faintly medical. I am afraid that there are too many things they can't cure; and that the cure is often worse than the disease; and I am afraid of the business of deciding whether a person, even myself, should live or die. This is a new phobia, you understand. This is the PTSD in action. This is the thing and the whole nature of the thing."[7] Risbridger was writing in March 2020 of how the experience of caring for a transplant patient had prepared her for the coronavirus pandemic: "The news was all test results, as my life had been for so long. . . . Every hand-washing guide made me wonder how there could be people who didn't *know* this; every mask badly fitted made me long to lean over and pinch the wire properly around the nose and ears. This was my world." I felt much the same through the pandemic, the social distancing, the long isolation. My learned responses jumped to attention, ready to plan, to advocate if Brad—an extremely high-risk patient—got sick, which, fortunately, hadn't come to pass as of this writing.

According to a 2005 study in the *American Journal of Respiratory and Critical Care Medicine*, caregivers who were deeply involved in end-of-life decisions or the death of a relative were more likely to experience aftereffects such as intrusive thoughts or flashbacks.[8] I thought, reading this, of the ending of Zora Neale Hurston's classic novel *Their Eyes Were Watching God*, which depicts the extreme trauma of Janie's efforts to care for her husband Tea Cake. She loves him deeply and cares for him tenderly in the later stages of rabies while also trying to get him medical help, but in the extremity of his disease she must shoot him in self-defense. Once she's alone, after she buries him and returns to her old home, "the day of the gun, and the bloody body, and the courthouse came and commenced to sing a sobbing sigh out of every corner in the room."[9] The all-encompassing return of her traumatic experience goes beyond a flashback—and her pain from caring for Tea Cake through severe, distressing illness is inextricable from the larger trauma. The lyrical description of the sobbing room illustrates, more vividly than a study can, how immersive post-trauma episodes can feel.

Grief like Janie's complicates the aftereffects of caregiving. These effects can last for months or years. A smaller 2012 study of relatives of ICU patients looked at family members three months after their ICU experience. That study found that the subjects were "at high risk for symptoms of PTSD, anxiety, and depression," with just under half experiencing intrusive thoughts, flashbacks, hyperarousal (in which the body's stress response goes into overdrive when thinking about the trauma), and nightmares.[10]

A well-known phenomenon in the caring professions, especially counseling, is "vicarious trauma," in which therapists and others take on the trauma of those they help.[11] The ongoing effects on caregivers may overlap with this category. A related, familiar term is compassion fatigue. Vicarious trauma differs from simple burnout, according to the American Counseling Association, in that it includes "tension and preoccupation," not just exhaustion and the inability to care further.[12]

Despite a few studies, little clinical attention has been devoted to how these related yet distinct conditions might affect family caregivers—one more sign of the degree to which the medical field takes caregivers for granted. A *New York Times* article by Judith Graham titled "For Some Caregivers, the Trauma Lingers,"[13] published in 2013 as part of the paper's New Old Age series, offers perspectives from various physicians, including one haunted by flashbacks to caregiving for her mother. Experts quoted in the piece, including a psychologist who's written on caregiving and a psychiatrist who treats caregivers, disagreed on whether there's enough evidence to conclude that caregiving can lead to post-traumatic stress. Ample anecdotal evidence, however, suggests caregivers can struggle after their duties end, whether or not the response is extreme enough to fit into a clinical diagnosis. That was certainly the case for me, and I found much to identify with in the more than 150 comments on Graham's piece, most from anguished caregivers sharing the challenges they've encountered.

Former caregiver Jennifer Levin, in a piece for the *Washington Post*, gives an account of picking up her mom from a routine health procedure and the beeps of medical monitors setting off "acute sensory flashbacks": her vision clouded and her body became overwhelmed by stress.[14] This reminded me acutely of Brad and me: neither of us, anymore, can abide a beeping machine, and we can't figure out how to turn off the beeping alerts of the end of our dishwasher and washing-machine cycles. When Brad was in the transplant unit, the sensors in the machine governing his IV tower would frequently trip, causing it to beep seemingly at random: air or a kink in the line, it would report, or a bag needed changing. Often it was a false alarm; other times the nurse needed to address the problem. It drove us both nuts, that beeping we couldn't fix—him more than me, since it was attached to his body. Our beeping dishwasher is far from the worst hangover of our years of medical crisis but it is a not-so-quiet daily reminder of it. All kinds of things can suddenly cause the hospital experience to rise up and distract me from the present moment: the smell of hand sanitizer, the sight of the blue Gatorade they brought Brad three times a day, news of the diagnosis of an acquaintance, or—the worst—actually setting foot in a hospital once again.

Levin also relates how stepping into a medical environment rocketed her back in time to the devastating experience of caring for her father as he declined from a degenerative brain disease. Levin's caregiving responsibilities differed from my own but her description of her reactions to reminders could have been mine: "I didn't realize at the time how traumatic these hospital visits were, or that their memories would haunt me. After he passed, classic PTSD symptoms, which included intrusive flashbacks, being 'dazed' when distressed, and avoiding medical settings reminiscent of his disease, recurred for a couple of years."

Moreover, as Levin points out, caregivers are often thrust into their roles suddenly or without their full consent, making the memories of caregiving all the more distressing. In the crisis of someone else's illness, caregivers tend simply to do what needs to be done, as Levin writes: "If you had told me when my father got ill that I could be at risk of developing PTS symptoms if I cared for him, my response probably would've been, 'I'll be fine.' Personal well-being isn't something caregivers think about much, perhaps because many don't have a choice about taking on this responsibility. I brushed aside any distress—such as panicking when my phone rang with an unknown number—as typical because, why wouldn't this be upsetting?" Besides, as Levin goes on to say, few caregivers can make time for mental healthcare and feelings of anxiety are usually an intrinsic part of caregiving. After all, if caregivers weren't anxious about our loved ones, why would we be giving up so much of our time and energy and resources to care for them?

AFRAID OF A DISASTER

I never suffered from particularly high levels of anxiety before Brad's illness. But once Brad was doing a little better and I could spare the time to take an assessment in my doctor's office, the results surprised me: how intense my anxiety was and how much it was interfering with my life. I was carrying on—I was always carrying on—but the effort was taking almost everything I had. For me the anxiety of crisis caregiving gave way directly to hypervigilance. One day, reading aloud to our younger daughter, I recognized precisely how I felt. I was like Miss Clavel, the long-suffering headmistress of the Parisian school in Ludwig Bemelmans's picture book *Madeline*. At the book's outset, Miss Clavel wakes up in the middle of the night knowing "something is not right," sitting bolt upright, worried about the children in her charge, and running "fast and faster" to their aid. It turns out Madeline has fallen ill and must go to the hospital, where she requires an appendectomy. Even after Madeline has recovered, though, Miss Clavel cannot rest: she wakes up in the night, hyperalert to the children's cries.

Caregiving and parenting through medical trauma have conditioned me, too, to expect further emergencies, to be ready at any moment to "run fast and faster" to someone's rescue, even when I don't really need to. I read the book as a child, and as a parent have read the book aloud to my daughters more times than I can count, but until Brad got sick I never gave a second thought to Miss Clavel. She is a sort of school Jacqueline-of-all-trades, mistress of none: she is the headmistress, apparently, but there is also a board of trustees, which seems excessive for a school with a mere twelve pupils, all of whom seem to stay there all the time and even go on international trips together. As a child I thought Miss Clavel was a nun—she wears a severe-looking habit—but as an adult I realized that nuns don't go by Miss Anything. I assumed that her garb must be some kind of French teacher situation I'm unfamiliar with but it actually more closely resembles that of a nurse. Besides, we never see any actual instruction happening in this school. Miss Clavel's role is more akin to nurse or nanny. She shepherds Madeline and eleven other girls around Paris in two straight lines; she worries they're unwell; she wakes up, terrified, in the middle of the night; she runs, "afraid of a disaster . . . fast and faster," with the illustrations showing her wheeling forward at an ever more impossible angle.[15]

Poor Miss Clavel. I get it, I really do. I, too, wake up in the middle of the night thinking something is not right. I have, lately, had children in my sole charge more than I expected. I have been traumatized by needing to call the doctor, suddenly, when I least expected to. I have a lot of problems with *Madeline* (it drives me a bit crazy that her name is neither spelled nor pronounced that way in French, though granted, it's an American picture book) and even more with its sequels, obvious money grabs with nonsensical story lines and verses that don't scan. But the verisimilitude of Miss Clavel is not among them. She is scarred, clearly, by being the sole adult in charge of children who need her, who get sick, for whose health she may be held responsible. She knows, as caregivers do, that often something will not be right, and she can't let it go.

I used to think that the middle-aged, anxious, worrywart women that all my friends' moms seemed to become were too fussy. Maybe, I realize now, they were realistic. Maybe they'd seen some shit I hadn't yet. Maybe they'd spent too long sleeping lightly, waiting to be awakened by an emergency great or small. Maybe I was sexist and ageist with the vast and unfightable sexism and ageism of our culture, which discounts the worries of middle-aged women, forgetting they are the ones who keep watch in the night. Forgetting, or collectively pretending we never knew, that the mythological Greek prophet Cassandra was right and disasters do come.

Once in the time before cancer, when our older daughter was six weeks old, Brad spent an entire day in bed, groaning. At first, as I could see nothing wrong with him and as our tiny daughter was crying, I was irritated. I thought he was being a baby about the pain he was claiming. It turned out to be appendicitis—something I finally guessed when he mentioned his stomach hurt on the lower right side, and I insisted he call the doctor to be seen immediately. The doctor sent him to the ER, my mom helped with the baby, and he had laparoscopic surgery. The hospital discharged him the next day. Later, when we could laugh about it, we called it his sympathetic pregnancy.

At the time we were both healthy. We'd always been young and healthy. An appendectomy seemed like a dramatic health crisis. Compared to his multiyear cancer ordeal an appendectomy now sounds like removing a splinter with tweezers. The appendectomy might be the least serious-seeming of all major surgeries, light enough to be the subject of a popular picture book like *Madeline*. One of the most memorable illustrations in the book is the eponymous heroine standing proudly post-appendectomy, feet planted, tummy outthrust, to show her classmates "the biggest surprise by far: on her stomach was a scar."

Madeline enjoys ten blissful days recovering in the hospital. She rests, she plays with a new dollhouse sent by her father and eats the candy he also sends, she enjoys thinking about the pictures on the ceiling formed by whimsically shaped cracks. The surgery gives Madeline cachet and her friends are envious. The jaunty bow on Madeline's head suggests her pride as she lifts her pajamas to reveal that scar on her round little belly.

My husband's stomach, too, used to be gently rounded, until in 2014 it wasn't; suddenly he was thin enough to have a six-pack, but instead of musculature on his flat abdomen we saw the formless bumps that turned out to be tumors. Something was not right. Our creeping feeling of dread increased until that night when he began coughing up blood, and I abruptly became a crisis caregiver. The terror of that night has stayed with me, as has the blur of wait-and-hurry-up hospital uncertainty that came after. The nineteen days Brad stayed with his collapsed lung were a far cry from the luxurious, restful ten-day stay Madeline got for her appendectomy. My husband's room had no dollhouse from Papa such as Madeline gets, nor flowers (not allowed on the oncology floor), nor candy.

During one of Brad's 2015 hospital stays for chemo, a different bout of coughing woke me up in the night. Lucy was nearly six at the time, old for croup, but I know the sound: the wheezing, painful, honking intake of breath betokens the narrowed, inflamed voice box, croup's hallmark. (Although most kids outgrow croup by age four or five, for some reason both of my daughters kept getting it well into the elementary school years, to the perennial surprise of their pediatrician.) It strikes only at night; during the day the child often seems fine. The best treatment is to get the child into cold air, which can work on the voice box to shrink its swelling, but cold air is hard to come by in Sacramento in July. A humidifier or a steamy shower is the second-best option, but it takes more time to work, and on this night my daughter was gasping out, "I . . . can't . . . breathe," in between squeaks. Something was not right.

My mother-in-law was staying with us so I didn't have to wake my older daughter—then 10—and drag her to the ER with me at 1 in the morning. I snatched up Lucy and, for the second time that summer, ran red lights en route to the emergency room. She got a breathing treatment and the steroid that, I'd learned, was the best way to prevent a worse attack on the second night of croup. (It's called dexamethasone, and Brad takes it now too, for his GvHD; in 2020, when it was reported that dexamethasone was one of the first treatments to show efficacy in severe cases of COVID-19, he joked that he'd need to refill his prescription immediately.) I lay on the uncomfortable extra bed the pediatric ER staff had wheeled in for the patient's tired mother and thought about the patient's father, sleeping eight floors up while he received a slow, four-day drip of chemotherapy, unaware our daughter and I were in the same building. Knowing I could be the last line of defense any time—that our child could gasp out that she couldn't breathe and it would be entirely my call as to what to do about it—only contributed to my growing, constant caregiver anxiety.

INVISIBLE SCARS

Brad bears both emotional and physical scars from his many treatments: biopsy marks on his back, the upper-chest bump where his port (a chest catheter implanted below the skin) still lies, a mark on his arm where his PICC (the central line used for his initial chemo) was inserted in 2015. My own scars from his treatment are less apparent, though there's no question that the stress of caregiving affected my body as well as my mind. My muscles got so tight I injured myself, snapping a knee so I could barely walk for days; my trapezius inflamed enough to immobilize my neck; my jaw grew sore from clenching. My hip flexors became tightly strung from sitting by a hospital bed, making my hips and lower back sore. I was always, always tired and couldn't sleep well. I gained weight, in part because I couldn't exercise much, in part because I soothed anxiety with food and drink. Sometimes a small (or not so small) treat was the only reliably pleasurable part of my day. Glynnis MacNicol, who writes extensively about caring for her mother through dementia and death in her memoir *No One Tells You This*, describes eating as solace in moments of caregiver guilt and strain: "The brief amount of pleasure the kids' chocolate Halloween candy brought me felt like the only comfort I could currently rely on. I decided I wasn't going to feel bad about this, even if it meant saying goodbye to my wardrobe. I was going to take the small bits of consolation where I could get them."[16] I made the same bargain, though I miss my old dresses and my old, pain-free body. I'm not sure which aches are from the six years I've aged while caregiving and which are from stress. I go after my muscles with a foam roller and excruciatingly try to grind out the physical effects of emotional strain. It helps, a little.

Most people probably don't notice that on plenty of days I feel like a wreck and like it's pointless to carry on. I always move forward anyway, usually wearing lipstick. But for years now if Brad oversleeps, or has a rusty smudge on his shirt that could be blood (but is probably food; when he was visually impaired, that happened all the time), or looks suddenly thinner than usual, I catch my breath and feel my adrenaline rise. My first thought is that something is not right.

The anxiety followed me everywhere, including on that writing trip I took to Mexico after the 2016 election. One night I woke and sat up like Miss Clavel. Something felt not right. In actuality, the drumbeat of the surf, which strengthened in the night, was what had awakened me. I left the sliding glass doors of my suite open to the breeze and slept with the mosquito netting gathered around me. The room was lovely: perfect for a couple, a little big for one person. It was clearly designed to signal to a couple on a romantic getaway that they should be having a lot of sex and napping. I did at least nap.

When I went uneasily back to sleep, I dreamed that my mother-in-law and my children and their friends had all arrived at the resort along with Brad, who had driven from the airport despite being unable to see properly. I had no idea what to do with him. He couldn't drink the water in Mexico. My younger daughter scribbled on walls (something she was far too old to do in reality) and fell off a balcony while playing on it—shades of Madeline, who in the second book of the series falls in the Seine while trying to scare Miss Clavel by walking tightrope-style on a bridge railing. In my dream I worried that the girls would be found by the people who work at the adults-only resort and we would all be kicked out. I worried how Brad would get home and wanted everyone to leave. I worried as much for myself—and the end of my vacation—as I did for them. It was only a dream, but it was a telling one about the degree to which caregiving has permanently changed me.

PRETTY TOUGH

As much as I could, I kept the extent of my caregiving scars to myself or shared them only with my therapist. In daily life, when people remembered to ask how I was doing, I would say I was fine or just shrug and say, "You know, hanging in there." I didn't need to do that too often; most people just asked about Brad. Similarly, Jennifer Levin says that her stock response to concerned queries was blunt: "I'll be fine." But the long-term reverberations of the trauma witnessed while caregiving can be intense, especially in extreme cases. Novelist Rebecca Makkai depicts such a case in *The Great Believers*. The novel cuts between the 1980s and the present, following two protagonists, both of whom assume caregiving roles they'd never anticipated: Yale Tishman, a gay man whose friends and ex-partner die of complications from AIDS and who contracts the disease himself, and Fiona Marcus, a straight woman who cares for her brother Nico and many others, including Yale. Fiona experiences lifelong trauma from the experience, which is all the worse because she refuses to confront it.[17] Dan Lopez's thoughtful review of the novel in the *L.A. Review of Books* points out that the novel is "recuperating the overlooked history of the women caretakers" of the AIDS epidemic. Lopez refers bluntly to Fiona's condition as PTSD.[18] Late in the novel, Fiona describes herself as "living for the past 30 years in a deafening echo."[19]

Shortly after Nico's death early in the AIDS crisis, Fiona becomes extremely close with Yale; as it happens, she's pregnant while caring for him and goes into labor at his hospital bedside. She doesn't want to leave him, and he has to tell her, mordantly, "'Maybe don't have your baby on the AIDS ward.'"[20] He also frets that his illness is retraumatizing her: "'Fiona, I hate that I'm putting you through this again. I'm worried what this is doing to you.' She rubbed her eyes, made a feeble effort to smile. 'I mean, it's bringing back memories. And it's killing me that it's you. You're my favorite person. But I'm pretty tough.'"[21] Yale dies, alone, while Fiona is giving birth on another floor. Tough or not, Fiona—after what she calls "the bloodbath of her twenties, after everyone she loved had died or left her"—is left emotionally wounded. She's especially stunted as a parent, unable to give her whole heart to her daughter, whose birth she associates with her guilt over Yale's death. That association leads to a lifelong rift between mother and child.

As I discussed in the previous chapter, children don't wait until after the challenges of caregiving to grow up. Now, as I grapple with the lingering emotional ripples of caregiving, my daughters continue to grow up without waiting for me to finish that fight. The problem with toughness is that a thick skin can mask deep difficulties. Like Fiona, I rarely cracked when Brad was ill. But since then I've needed significant therapy. Being in a hospital brings up feelings of mild panic, but even more so, a prolonged groan from Brad will often cause me to sit up straight and peer at him intently, like some kind of medically trained prairie dog. Since he groans frequently (even several years after transplant he is in pain most of the time), I'm always on high alert.

For at least a couple of years during and following Brad's treatment, I awoke regularly around 3 a.m., a difficult time. I have the luxury of taking half a Xanax (a benzodiazepine used as an anti-anxiety medication) when I really can't get back to sleep. I also started taking Prozac for a time. Miss Clavel had none of these aids; all she could do, it seems, was to affix her headdress and run fast and faster down the stairs to check on those twelve little girls sleeping in two straight lines. At first, when my doctor suggested an antidepressant, I said no. Prozac, I thought, wouldn't ameliorate the condition causing my anxiety and depression, which was strictly situational. But I yielded when I realized in shock that on the anxiety scale I'd marked "more than half the time" for nearly all of the questions about how anxiety was affecting me. Now I'm not so resistant to medication, which did help. It was also easier for me to get a prescription for an ongoing antidepressant than for occasional anxiety relief like Xanax or Ativan: my doctor had offered me eight pills of either of those and said it was a three-month supply—benzos are highly addictive. Brad, though, as a cancer patient, routinely received a thirty-day, thirty-pill prescription of Xanax with unlimited refills. He gave me the occasional pill as a workaround since I had more anxiety than two or three doses a month could manage.

My fear of Brad's imminent death has faded as his condition has improved but reminders like those beeping machines—or, recently, another diagnosis of aggressive lymphoma in our extended family—still give me a tense, uneasy feeling. My continuing anxiety has been driven by regret as well as legitimate medical concern. It's not comfortable to recall my first response to that crisis: irritation. I flinched when I watched the Netflix series *The Crown* and it opened with King George VI's bloody coughing fit—a sign of rapidly fatal lung cancer that reminded me pointedly of Brad's first hospitalization. I could watch the later episodes—in which the king has gruesome surgery and eventually dies—with equanimity, but I had to pause the video after the initial shock of that cough. In early 2020, when any cough became a terrifying potential indicator of COVID-19, my response became even more exaggerated. It didn't help that at the time the pandemic was hitting California, Brad had an apparently unrelated lung infection that the doctors couldn't quite diagnose. Even though the COVID-19 cough was always described as drier than what Brad presented and he didn't have the telltale fever, my heart pounded every time I heard him emit a wet, gurgling rasp.

Somewhere deep inside I'm quicker to see catastrophe coming. I'm less trusting, less patient, blunter—not just with medical personnel but with family and even friends. I'm frustrated by Brad's limitations even as I know I ought to be grateful he's alive. I'm irritable and snappish sometimes with his minor symptoms. I've struggled to adjust to whatever we could call the new normal. Though the intensity of these aftereffects has faded with time, they still linger for me as a caregiver and even more so for Brad as a now chronically ill patient, making it hard to repair our lives together in the wake of our extended crisis.

NINE

THE AFTERMATH

Rebuilding from Caregiving

When I sat down to write this chapter, it was five years to the day since Brad asked me if he should go to the doctor because of the weird lumps on his jawline and I said yes. I remember the feeling of unease I had then but also the innocence, the near-total failure to sense impending disaster. In those five years, I feel like I've aged fifteen years and he's aged fifty. He's not sick now but he's not well either: he lives in an uncertain world of chronic illness. (He was at the hospital for treatment when I wrote this paragraph.) We've had to navigate a new narrative of disability as we've emerged uncertainly from the whirlwind of cancer treatment. I don't really know if I'm still a caregiver. Do I count? The kind of caregiving I'm doing now is hard to define or explain to an outsider. Sometimes I wonder if I'm doing anything at all, even as I have to urge him to call the doctor about a new symptom or intervene to stop Brad from riding his bike to an X-ray appointment when he has suspected pneumonia. There's been no formal end to my caregiving life, though its demands have eased considerably. Still, I hardly know how to go back to a sense of myself as a person living for myself—much less as a partner in a marriage to someone who has been changed even more than I have.

What does it mean to be a former caregiver, and how do we go back to a regular marriage when everything about our roles was so completely changed by Brad's sickness? The postcancer period of our lives has been marked by setbacks and uncertainty, both in Brad's health and our relationship. When the coronavirus pandemic struck, for instance, our old patterns reared up immediately, with me worrying about him and strategizing about what I would do if he contracted it. I wasn't alone; it was a challenging time for caregivers everywhere, especially sandwiched ones responsible for an elderly and vulnerable parent, as writer Sarah Stankorb vividly illustrated in a piece on caregiving during coronavirus for the *Lily*.[1] (It took several weeks before it occurred to me that I also ought to worry about myself getting it.) Still, I don't make his medical appointments or manage his medications anymore. After four eye surgeries he can see well enough to drive again. In a fight not long ago he said I'm not really his caregiver anymore, and that's true. But everything about our relationship is still conditioned by his illness and my once—and probably future—caregiving role. In the culture of cancer the phase we're in now is the one called the New Normal, a phrase that's become hackneyed but sums it up as well as any. Brad struggles with his new role as, essentially, a professional patient. I struggle to get back to work and marriage and regular life.

Rebuilding our lives after the deep trauma of his illness hasn't been easy. Despite the easy "new normal" shorthand, there aren't many real, honest models for how to live after severe illness, for either partner. If caregivers are all but invisible in our culture, those of us who are living in the shadowy, uncertain world after caregiving are not just unseen; nobody even recognizes our situation as a real phenomenon. I've struggled to feel like myself again in this ambiguous after. Sometimes I almost miss the stress of the periods when Brad was actively, critically ill, because at least then I understood why I was so down all the time.

AFTER THE CHAINS

What happens to caregivers after the direct, hands-on caregiving ends? It varies tremendously, according to the situation. Often the care recipient has died—though, as Arthur Kleinman notes in *The Soul of Care*, "Care does not end with death but involves actively caring for memories."[2] Sometimes they have recovered. Sometimes caregivers leave or hand off responsibilities to another family member. And often the situation isn't clear-cut. Sandwiched caregivers will find that some duties go on when others are relinquished. Family caregivers of, say, a parent may trade off primary responsibility with siblings, and thus get breaks but not a permanent respite. Sometimes caregivers may become ill or in need themselves, leading to reciprocal care or an entirely new situation. Sometimes, as in my case, the crisis becomes less acute but the care recipient has ongoing needs. For others, there's a short, sharp shock of crisis caregiving—say, when a spouse has major surgery—that quickly fades back to normalcy.

In *Anne's House of Dreams*, Leslie Moore's caregiving duties end in a far more dramatic fashion than most—but still held meaningful resonance to me. In a plot twist that frees Leslie, Anne's husband, Gilbert, a doctor, has read about a seemingly miraculous brain surgery that can restore Dick's senses.[3] Gilbert and Anne have their first marital disagreement about the surgery. Anne knows Leslie would be even more miserable if her abusive husband were restored. Gilbert, however, feels it's his duty to tell Leslie that Dick could be cured. Leslie grimly agrees to the operation—only to find that the man to whom she has been laboriously tending for years is in fact her husband's cousin, "George Moore of Nova Scotia, who, it seems, always resembled him very strikingly. Dick Moore died of yellow fever thirteen years ago in Cuba."[4]

Montgomery piles up reason after reason why this mistaken identity could have gone unnoticed: Leslie, younger than her husband, never met the look-alike cousin; the two men "both had that queer freak of eyes—one blue and one hazel."[5] Dick and George are double cousins—their fathers are brothers; their mothers, identical twins—who sailed to Cuba on the same ship. Dick happened to die after giving George letters and his watch to take to Leslie; George, after his injury, happened to be found, with no other identifying information, by seafaring Captain Jim, who knew Dick on Prince Edward Island. The Captain, fooled by the watch and letters, brought "Dick" home to Leslie. The entire community attributed differences in "Dick" to his accident.

After the discovery of the mistaken identity, Leslie's story transforms into pure romance. George is transferred to the care of a long-lost sister. Leslie has fallen in love with a writer who vacationed on the island and the two are free to marry. The story ends happily. Anne says to Leslie: "'Your chain is broken—there is no cage.'" When Leslie's suitor, hearing of her freedom, returns to the island to court her, Anne tells her: "'Take off your tragic airs, my dear friend, and fold them up and put them away in lavender. You'll never need them again.'"[6]

Perhaps she won't. But the truth about caregiving is that it doesn't set anyone free, not easily. Miracle cures rarely snap a patient back to health, much less reveal that oh, oops, he's not your husband after all and you're free to walk away. For many caregivers, their duties end only with the death of their beloved, a fact that necessarily comes with loss and grief and sometimes a guilty, perhaps half-smothered relief. For others—for me—the burden slowly, gradually lightens as the sick person recovers, but it leaves behind a life changed utterly. In my case I was left feeling more alone than ever before: alienated from many friends, bereft of many former pursuits, my husband a different-seeming man.

As fairy-tale-like as Leslie's sudden freedom is, it does hold a pointed metaphor. In positing that the person you care for is not the person you knew before the illness, Montgomery's story reveals a deeper, deeply painful truth. In fundamental ways, I haven't been caring for the husband I once knew. Brad is different—changed physically and in personality. His outlook, his interests, his hopes are different than they were before his diagnosis; mine are too. As he has improved, both of us have emerged, like Leslie, out of the cages his illness built.

Whatever the reason for the end of care, the literature around caregiving has begun to recognize that period as a distinct stage, though there's still a long way to go in supporting caregivers after their duties end. Much of the advice for the post-caregiving stage is practical: pick up old hobbies, call up old friends, go to a movie since you have the time now. To my mind such advice leaves out the emotional side of a time marked by depression, post-trauma symptoms (as discussed in the previous chapter), and profound feelings of loss, often alongside but distinct from grief over the care recipient's death.

I've seen better, more comprehensive approaches recently on major caregiver resource websites such as AARP, the Caregiver Space, and the Family Caregiver Alliance, all of which offer pages discussing issues that arise after caregiving responsibilities end. There's even a $20, self-led, six-week webinar course available from the website CareGiving.com, called "Beginning Again after Caregiving Ends," with the stated objective: "At the end of our course, you will feel comforted about your past, feel confident about your future and feel ready to begin your present." The modules move from a first class on closing out the experience (with such topics as "reconciling resentments") to week six, "Share" ("Your life; your dreams").[7] Site founder Denise M. Brown developed the course to address what she saw as a gap in resources for caregivers; she calls the post-caregiving phase "Godspeed Caregiving" and includes a PDF of a book, *After Caregiving Ends, a Guide to Beginning Again*, with registration.

Brown may have been a pioneer in developing a post-caregiving resource, but her website is no longer alone in the field. Such resources tend to offer similar-sounding themes. It's neatly summed up in a tip sheet by social worker Donna Schempp, from the Caregiver Alliance, "When Caregiving Ends": "Caregivers set their own lives aside to care for someone else [and then] have to figure out what to do with their lives now. There is no preparation for this transition. Generally you are so busy caregiving, and life changed so long ago, that there has not been time nor energy or even the psychological will to think about what comes next."[8] Or, as Mary Helen Berg writes in the *AARP Bulletin*, "Caring for another adult . . . can be demanding to the point that caregivers put much of their own lives on hold. When those duties suddenly end, the caregiver is left not only grieving but also processing new emotions about their own station in life."[9]

They're also left processing a complex, highly individual blend of feelings: grief, relief (both for oneself and on behalf of a suffering loved one) or even exhilaration, guilt or shame (often about the relief), exhaustion, regret, profound emptiness, anger, resentment, loneliness. In cases where there's no clear endpoint to caregiving, like mine, these emotions can sit alongside the need to carry on in a relationship to a care recipient who may be profoundly changed by severe illness, as Brad was.

For other caregivers, circumstances like these combine in vastly different ways. When the stress of intense caregiving ends with the death of the care recipient, the caregiver's grief may be complicated and exacerbated. A new project begins of caring for the person after death, from the immediate questions of handling the body to the longer work of all of the business matters brought on by a death. After my mother's suicide, my brother and I were the co-executors of her will, and the long project of shutting up the shop of a whole life dragged on through months and years. As hard as it was, it can provide closure. Calling every bureaucracy

I'd ever dealt with during my mom's illness to complete the work of wrapping up her life sharply delineated an end point. It also kept me moving through a period of shock. Both then and, at some points, in caring for Brad, I felt like if I stopped to cry or grieve or even think, I might never get back up again. But after the busy time ends, all that emotion remains and has to be worked through.

Glynnis MacNicol, who writes about caring for her mother long-distance through a steep decline into dementia in *No One Tells You This*, gives a memorable self-portrait of emptiness and loss after caregiving.[10] MacNicol—who, in the period that she chronicles, also happens to be turning forty, questioning her single and childless state, and overextending herself nurturing several friends and family members as the crisis with her mother comes to a head—feels painfully empty after settling her mother in a care home and helping to sell her parents' home. "Just like that, it seemed, everything had let up. . . . As my mother might have said, 'giddy Fortune's furious fickle wheel' had turned and taken with it many of the responsibilities and concerns that had dominated my last year and a half. It should all have been a relief, but instead I felt conflicted by the shift. To suddenly find myself unnecessary on all fronts was jarring and made me feel strangely disposable. And what was I now supposed to do with all the freedom?"[11] MacNicol's feelings are exacerbated by her sense that she and her mother never really quite understood each other; she's experiencing complicated grief for a mother who has not yet died but is nevertheless lost to her.

MacNicol questions whether she did enough to ensure that her mother was well cared for, and she grieves their relationship even as she feels like she should do more with her newfound freedom: "I was wide open. But before I could stop it, into that empty space, like an emotional squatter, crept all the grief and sadness I'd held at bay. The tears I'd choked back the day we'd left my mother in the nursing home, and all the days I'd left her since. The overwhelming loss of standing by while her mind evaporated. . . . Knowing the inevitable ending that was coming."[12] That feeling—of finally having the sadness flood in only once there's time for it—is one I know only too well.

Louisa May Alcott paints a sorrowful, familiar portrait of Jo March in the wake of her sister Beth's death in *Little Women*. Jo has been "wrapped up" in Beth's care, and now that Beth is gone she faces the isolation of mourning and a painful loss of purpose. She had promised Beth that she will look after their aging parents, with whom the sisters had both lived in the family home, but "when [Beth's] helpful voice was silent, the daily lesson over, the beloved presence gone, and nothing remained but loneliness and grief, then Jo found her promise very hard to keep." Her sorrow is exacerbated in these "dark days" by the loss of the work of caregiving, and she has no sense of what to replace it with: "where in all the world could she 'find some useful, happy work to do' that would take the place of the loving service which had been its own reward?"[13] Jo, like Jane Eyre before her, finds caregiving intrinsically rewarding—an assertion that may, in this autobiographical novel, reflect Alcott's grief about the loss of her own sister, as well as a certain conformity to the gender norms of the novel's day. In her grief Jo feels despair when she thinks of "spending all her life in that quiet house."

As Jo learns it can be challenging to reconnect with the world after the isolation of caregiving, a subject that MacNicol also explores. When her mother dies, several of MacNicol's friends offer to fly to Toronto for the funeral. MacNicol, caught off guard by the outpouring of support, brushes them off: "I was so accustomed to doing things on my own, it didn't occur to me that this would be any different. I thought I was prepared. . . . I didn't realize what a terrible error I had made until the morning of the funeral."[14] At the funeral itself, MacNicol says she feels "like a ship being violently tossed on the ocean with no anchor, no port, exposed."[15]

NO ANCHOR, NO PORT

During the years of my caregiving responsibilities, I started to feel unmoored from the most basic facts of my life. My marriage felt less like ballast keeping me on an even keel and more like a weight so heavy it could sink me. Our home felt not like a safe harbor but like a maelstrom of responsibilities and painful emotions, with reminders everywhere of the storm we were living through.

Maybe it's no accident that the hobby I took up to get back into the swing of life when the grip of caregiving relaxed (see, I've tried to follow the well-meaning advice!) has been rowing on a crew. There's been something comforting about setting off in a tiny low boat with eight other people, surrendering to their rhythm while a coxswain steers us all, then returning safe to dock as the sun is rising. All you have to think about is keeping your own oar handle steady and in time with everyone else. The only weight you need to pull is your own. It's surprising, once you think about it, how many idioms of daily life are metaphors borrowed from the language of boats and ships. I find it much easier to keep an even keel in a boat designed for that purpose than in the wobbly realities of daily life.

Part of what makes it hard to keep moving forward is the degree to which physical reminders of Brad's illness still pervade our lives. One weekend when he was suffering from both a sore throat and a GvHD flare-up, I was puttering around reorganizing a utility cupboard full of jumbled light bulbs, batteries, laundry detergent, and the like. Deep on the shelf of batteries was a goldenrod-yellow 9-volt, alone in its own small plastic bag. I picked it up and recognition jolted me: this was the last battery left from those huge packs that had been delivered to us weekly when Brad needed IV nutrition. I recalled that senior physician who waved off the challenge of hooking up the pump and then took a moment to think with relief of how much easier Brad's care had become since then. But even though things are easier, the feeling of responsibility has lingered, like that little yellow battery.

During Brad's long convalescence, he slept in our basement guest room, and he still sets up there for the night whenever he's feeling especially poorly or having trouble sleeping, conditions that also cause him to withdraw further into himself. Recently he's had to relocate from our shared bedroom with bouts of pneumonia and the itchiness of a skin rash caused by GvHD, both of which interfered with his sleep. He moved downstairs during the coronavirus pandemic as well, the better to stay away from me in case I was an asymptomatic carrier. We're fortunate to have so much space for ourselves but sometimes I wonder whether that space saved our marriage or widened the gulf still between us. Truth be told, I sleep a little better in a bed by myself anyway.

At times, feelings of profound loneliness within the marriage have brought me to the brink of ending it. A lot of things kept me from leaving: the thought of our girls, deep senses of guilt and responsibility, the thought of how hard people (even readers of this book, I imagined) would judge me, and—a painful truth—the presentiment that a separation or divorce would just be another hard project of emotional and logistical work I'd have to do.

STILL MARRIED TO A STRANGER

Over more than five years of diagnosis, treatment, and chronic illness, Brad's appearance changed dramatically, many times. His body became strange to me, far more so than when I posted that joking "married to a stranger!" status on Facebook. He's even genetically different, with his brother's DNA in his blood. His corneas come from two unknown donors. In his two cataract surgeries, the lenses of his eyes were replaced with strangely glittery artificial ones.

Normally we take the looks of those we love for granted. Over the past twenty years, Brad and I have of course aged. But to each other, we always looked about the same—until his cancer diagnosis. Brad and I met when I was twenty-three, and we are solidly in middle age now. The devastation of the body is what cancer does best, and that shows up in PET scans, on hairless heads, in clouded eyes, in loss of muscle or water-ballooning of fluid or pallor of skin. The scorched-earth campaign of transplant made Brad all but unrecognizable. Bedridden for four months, he lost muscle mass until his legs became thin, trembling sticks; they are still painfully skinny. Our care workers said they would not have known he was the same man as the robust, bearded person smiling in the family photos on our walls.

My husband's changed body is practically a map of his illness and the scars it left. Even his smell changed: because of radiation he no longer sweats much, and so his pheromones have faded, replaced by the ever-present odor of hand sanitizer. It probably hasn't helped our physical relationship that we've often been in separate bedrooms during his recovery. I lost my sex drive almost entirely during Brad's major hospitalization, but later terribly missed physical intimacy.

I can't decide if it's completely unsurprising or a sign of a deep character flaw in me—or both—that I'm not attracted to him the way I was before, though it feels cruel to say it. Seeing how ill he was in the transplant unit was a kind of trauma. I've heard some men say seeing their wives give birth can temporarily dampen desire; seeing my husband's body close to death, incontinent, swollen, and helpless, had a similar effect on me, one I hope will someday fade.

Sexuality requires—at least for me—a small space in which to be carefree. This is hard to come by as a full-time caregiver, and hard to create even in the post-caregiving phase if reminders of the illness linger. A small, painful scene showing one impact of care responsibilities on sexuality comes up in the love-it-or-hate-it movie *Love Actually*, in which Laura Linney's character is hyper-responsible for her institutionalized brother. When she's finally about to get together with the man she's had a crush on for years, her brother calls, she picks up, and the possibility of connection and sex are crushed.

There are few depictions of how a sex life can change after caregiving but I was moved by one in Mary Beth Keane's recent novel *Ask Again, Yes*—a tender examination of marriage, caregiving, and forgiveness. The novel's primary caregiver figure is Lena, whose husband, Francis Gleeson, has been shot in the face by a neighbor and undergoes a long, grueling recovery. His face changes radically and he loses an eye, but the key to their loss of a sex life seems to be Lena's changed feeling for him. Although the narration rotates among the major characters, we unfortunately see Lena's caregiving only from the point of view of other people—specifically Francis, who tries to understand the loss of their sexual relationship even as he is silently distressed by it: "She'd gotten so used to caring for him and worrying about him that it reminded him of what she'd been like when the girls were toddlers," he thinks. The one time they do have sex after his injury, he can tell "she'd done it only for him and not at all for herself." Finally, he understands that "she'd gotten used to being the caretaker and him the patient. She no longer went pale every time he made for the stairs, but she'd placed him in a category alongside the girls, the mortgage—another thing to worry about."[16] Even as I identified deeply with Lena's situation, I wished we could have heard her character's thoughts on these issues directly. Omitting her point of view from the narration struck me as a further erasure of caregivers as anything other than angels of service.

Being a patient for a prolonged period of time changes a person. I sense changes in Brad, particularly in his passivity and his cognition, that I'm not sure he recognizes in himself—or that many others see. He seems more like an older person: slower, more tentative, and more rigid. The need to roll with changes in family life with kids (especially, I find, on carpool days) throws him badly. Sometimes it feels like Brad has aged rapidly into a world I'm not ready to be in yet, a world of fragile health and old age: of querulousness, of hesitation, of fussing, of moving slowly. I'm not yet fifty, and I'm not ready to settle into that frail world. I don't love thinking or admitting that but I find myself frequently locked in frustration and unsure how to change it. It often ends up being easier to do things myself than to explain them to my husband. Our interests, too, have diverged. After the isolation of his illness, all I really want to do now is to get outdoors, to be physically active. If I had my way I'd be rowing most days and backpacking, trekking to a swimming hole, or camping in the summer. Outdoor adventures aren't possible for Brad, who must take with him dozens of medications, whose energy levels are unpredictable, and who is medically immune suppressed, making all but the tamest outings unwise.

I feel an emotional distance between us every day. I know Brad loves me but I rarely feel a sense of him reaching out to me, or, for that matter, to anybody. We are both home most days, yet we interact little. Many books I've read on caregiving talk about how the experience can bring the caregiver and recipient together, fostering closeness. For Brad and me this was true at first, but over time our experiences diverged so greatly it had the opposite effect. The worlds of the isolation unit in the hospital and the busy life of childrearing and running a household were so far apart. Even long after his return to the household, however, the question of how to run it has continued to be a source of conflict. We've both had to compromise our approaches to emotional labor and mental load in attempts to build a newly equitable marriage. The results have been mixed. I still feel put upon a lot of the time; Brad still feels defensive and like he's trying his best a lot of the time. Maybe he is. Maybe I need to lower my expectations some more. Some days are fine. But other days I don't know how much lower my expectations can get.

AMBIGUITY, THE NEW NORMAL

I don't have a nice neat place to end my story of caregiving. The situation, our new normal, continually shapes our marriage. I don't know where we'll end up five years from now, or even a year from now: Brad could get sick again at any time. I'm braced to jump back into full-time caregiving—a concern that became especially acute during the coronavirus pandemic. As the virus hit the US in the late winter of 2020 and we faced the truth of Brad's extreme vulnerability, I at first thought of how all of my practice in caregiving had prepared me to care for him and advocate for him. Then I realized that—because of the strict limits on hospital visitors and caregivers as part of COVID-19 precautions—there was no chance I would even get in the door. It was a terrifying thought, both for our personal situation and more broadly for the thousands of COVID patients who've had to face severe illness alone.

· · ·

I never expected to find myself, in my late forties, worn out from caring for an ill husband, unsure whether I have the fortitude to soldier on if or when he faces another health crisis, uncertain about how life will unfold as the world endures a global health crisis. Our family's path through the continuing pandemic is uncertain as well. As I write this in the summer of 2020, restrictions on businesses and public life are loosening—even though cases are beginning to spike again—but for Brad's protection we have to be cautious about engaging with the wider world until there's a vaccine or effective public health measures. Strangely, in some ways this quieter season—when the whole outside world has entered the kind of isolation that we endured after Brad's transplant—has brought us a little closer together. Maybe it's that the pace of my life has slowed to match Brad's. Sharing small joys like family trivia quizzes (we take turns making up the questions) and the odd walk around the neighborhood has given us more common ground. At this writing, the big picture is still anxiously uncertain. I don't know if we'll be able to send the kids to school next year (or if school will resume) or how long our family isolation will have to last. But I know I'll keep going; I have to. And meanwhile some of the aftereffects of my caregiving continue, draining me as they have drained so many others. For me and for millions of my fellow family caregivers enduring the pressures and fallout of supporting the people we love, the work is unsustainable. That's why we must, as a society, find better ways to care for one another.

CONCLUSION

DAMAGE CONTROL

How to (Really) Help Caregivers

We are all born needing care, and most of us die needing it too. Nearly all of us will also need help when we're ill along the way. It's not weak or unusual to want and need tending, despite what the American culture of individualism—and the laws and policies that reinforce it—might have us all think. The care we want and need in illness or other troubles can take many forms, whether it's as small as asking for tissues and spicy soup when battling a sinus infection or as all-encompassing as the kind of support Brad needed. Somebody has to provide that care, and odds are that the people who do the job, being human, will also need care for themselves, and so on and so on. How can we make it easier, as a society, to ensure that everybody gets the care they need?

There are plenty of well-intentioned caregiver resources out there to tell us what the solutions are. As we've seen, however, many put the onus right back on the already overburdened caregiver to arrange for their own self-care. Solutions involving respite care or the like are profoundly inaccessible for the millions of caregivers who lack financial resources to dip into, family or social ties to draw on, or the luxury of even an hour of free time. As I've said, I was more privileged than most, and I was able to do most of that. But—as I often thought about pregnancy—even an easy version of caregiving isn't easy.

The issue—which I think is the case with so many of our big problems in the United States—is that all of these measures offer small-scale, individual solutions to large-scale, systemic shortcomings. The challenges of caregiving arise not because individual families have foolishly failed to set themselves up better to do it. They exist because our society consistently devalues care and does little or nothing to support it. Much as climate change won't be solved by me getting my kids to use reusable snack bags, the crisis in care can't be addressed by any number of massages for individuals. (Not to pick on massages, which I love—or on my kids, who are getting better about single-use plastics.) For systemic problems we need systemic solutions, which involve a sea change in cultural attitudes and bold, ambitious plans to change laws and policies.

WHERE WE ARE NOW

Care may be a universal need but it's not always a hot-button issue for policymakers, for whom the issue is often invisible. Valuing care isn't merely a matter of policy—but it is a necessary precondition for creating good policy. The work of caregivers, as economically important as it is, is still dismissed or, often, unseen.

That may be starting to change, says Janet Kim, the communications director for Caring Across Generations: "Even in the current political climate, we can get policymakers to acknowledge the problem. But they get stuck in the details of the solution. The challenge lies in getting leaders to see the need for transformational solutions, and not settling for the incremental or piecemeal." Advocacy from ordinary people, caregivers among them, is critical, she says: "The political landscape needs to change but the good news is that we're starting to see more and more people from the grassroots demanding it."[1] In a 2019 poll, Caring Across Generations found that four out of five respondents—regardless of political affiliation—would support universal family care as a new federal program, which citizens would pay into and then be able to withdraw from when they need long-term care and other supports. The organization advocates for what it calls "a strong care infrastructure that can meet the needs of 21st century families,"[2] calling it Universal Family Care. The program, as outlined in a 2019 report from the nonpartisan nonprofit National

Academy of Social Insurance (which discloses on its website that it received support for the report from Caring Across Generations), would integrate various care programs and needs into a single state-based social insurance program. This program would include early childhood education, childcare, paid medical and family leave, and long-term care services and supports.[3] Such a system would enable all families and caregivers to draw on social insurance for the rapidly growing costs of long-term care, supports for in-home care, caregiver leaves from work, and other needs. Interestingly, Kim told me that although support for universal childcare wanes after voters are out of their childrearing years, support for long-term care and caregiver support is high across all age groups—perhaps reflecting the fact that so many people of all ages have seen a beloved grandparent or other older relative in need of care.

When I spoke to Jenna Gerry, a senior staff attorney in the Work and Family Program of the San Francisco–based nonprofit Legal Aid at Work (LAAW), she told me that in her experience legislators and staff tend to be more interested in parental leave than in caregiving—possibly because of the obvious "aww" factor of parental bonding with tiny babies. "What's critical is finding a way to really make [caregiving] an issue people care about," Gerry said. "It's a crisis that's coming, but when you're talking about parental leave, people home in on that and new babies. I've found it challenging at times to get that same level of interest in working for policy change around caregiving."[4]

Kim also acknowledges the challenges, especially with legislators who oppose expanding any social programs, and says that Caring Across Generations promotes a twofold strategy: "In the design of our policy, at its core Universal Family Care is built on a social insurance model which has proven to garner and sustain bipartisan support and be politically durable," she says. "But it's also important to appeal to care as a universal issue, which legislators must also know in their personal lives. We've almost universally been faced with caregiving challenges. The key is connecting our individual experiences and struggles and expanding them out to the experiences and struggles of our families, out to our communities—and realizing that it's a systemic failure, not an individual one."

The benefits of such a program are obvious but sometimes hard to visualize. Writer and caregiver Aisha Adkins—who founded Our Turn 2 Care, an organization that aims to connect marginalized millennial caregivers—brings them into focus in a recent essay, published on *Blavity*, about the challenges she faces as a younger Black caregiver: difficulties finding and keeping a job given the demands of her mother's care, damaged credit, health effects due to stress. Adkins advocates passionately for Universal Family Care, which would benefit her and all caregivers: "Imagine what it would be like to take the necessary time to care for a loved one without having to pick, choose and pray about which bill to pay and which prescription to go without? What if you didn't have to panic every month when you have to decide between rent and medication, lights and car note, or healthy food and affordable food?"[5]

At the federal level there's currently little support for caregivers, which means there's a significant opportunity for improvement and systemic change. The Family and Medical Leave Act, passed in 1993, guarantees twelve weeks of unpaid leave for family care to government and school workers, as well as employees of private companies with fifty or more employees. To be eligible for FMLA, workers must have been with their employer for a year in which they worked more than 1,250 hours—slightly more than half time.[6]

Those strictures leave out a lot of workers—and the fact that the leave is unpaid makes it impossible for many to take advantage of this bare-minimum benefit even if they are eligible. As Anne Boyer points out in *The Undying*, family leave also limits the help available to the ill: "In the United States, if you aren't someone's child, parent, or spouse, the law allows no one else guaranteed leave from work to take care of you. If you are loved outside the enclosure of family, the law doesn't care how deeply—even with all the unofficialized love in the world enfolding you, if you need to be cared for by others, it must be in stolen slivers of time."[7] Expanding leave policies to more people would benefit care recipients and caregivers alike, allowing for wider care networks to work together and easing the burden on any one primary caregiver. As noted in chapter 6, the coronavirus pandemic—which exposed our society's considerable fault lines and gaps around issues of care—prompted the creation of a limited and often hard-to-access provision for paid leave, but as of this writing it was still unclear whether that expansion would lead to lasting change.

There's a patchwork of state policies that supplement FMLA and extend assistance to caregivers. As of the end of 2019 paid family and medical leave was available in only eight states, plus the District of Columbia: Rhode Island, New Jersey, California, New York, Washington, Massachusetts, Connecticut, and Oregon.[8] Oregon's law, passed at the end of 2019 but not set to take effect until 2023, includes pay replacement up to 100 percent as well as job protections, and notably includes an expanded definition of family, including close relationships "by affinity." According to Kim, Caring Across Generations is optimistic about meaningful legislation emerging over the next few years to support care in several states, among them Michigan, Minnesota, Illinois, California, and possibly New Mexico.

New laws in my home state of California would build on our existing caregiving leave policies, which are already some of the best in the US: they include both partial wage replacement for up to six weeks and job protection for up to twelve weeks. Yet these benefits are often challenging at best to access, with difficult-to-navigate paperwork and gaps in eligibility that keep many workers from using their rights to the fullest. LAAW, which helped to advocate for paid family leave in 2002, summarizes California caregivers' rights and benefits in a dense fact sheet and operates a work and family help line that gets about one thousand calls per year.[9] Sharon Terman, director of LAAW's Work and Family Program, told me, "The programs can be complicated and difficult to navigate. As an example, people would assume that you would be able to take advantage of paid family leave without risking your job, but you have to qualify for both job protection and wage replacement. The requirements are different, and that causes a huge amount of confusion for people. It's a very stressful thing. To have programs that aren't easy to access and navigate is a huge barrier."[10] The nature of caregiving creates additional challenges, says LAAW attorney Jenna Gerry: "Because of the unique nature of caregiving, compared to [parental] bonding, it's much more complicated to access your rights. Caregiving is often more intermittent and requires more paperwork." Caregivers often tend to need a day here and a day there, rather than the continuous chunk of time that typically comprises parental bonding. In part because of such challenges, according to Gerry, only 10 percent of paid family leave claims in California are for caring for an ill family member.

Many Americans assume that Medicare will fill care gaps for elderly people who can't afford long-term care, but Medicare addresses only strictly medical needs—not care assistance such as residential care, retrofitting a shower, or paying home-care attendants so that a family caregiver can go to work. (Medicaid does cover nursing-home costs for low-income seniors.) As we've seen, long-term care looks set to be a pressing social issue in the decades ahead. Some states whose populations have aged more rapidly than others, such as Hawaii and Vermont, have proposed or implemented innovative solutions, such as long-term care benefits programs.[11] Hawaii offers a program called the Kupuna Caregivers Program, which was created in 2017 and provides up to $70 per day—which can cover such costs as adult day care and in-home support services—for those who work outside the home and are also providing long-term care to an elderly family member. (*Kupuna* means "elder" or "grandparent" in Hawaiian.) According to Caring Across Generations, which advocates for expanding the program, "Not only is this investment going to make the daily lives of family caregivers in Hawaiʻi better, it also is an inspiring step forward in addressing the economic [penalties] the 44 million family caregivers across the country can incur, especially for women who take on this role."[12]

In 2019, the state of Washington became the first to implement publicly funded long-term care with its Long-Term Care Trust Act.[13] The new law provides for a public fund—which residents must pay into for a minimum of ten years—that elderly or disabled Washington residents can tap, up to $100 per day, to assist with activities of daily living or other care needs.[14] The lifetime cap on funds, however, is $36,500—or one year of the maximum daily benefit—an amount that those with high care needs may run through quickly. The new fund is complemented by a distinctive professional training program for in-home caregivers, run by the Service Employees International Union. This program increases Washington residents' access to well-trained home-care workers.[15] Home-care workers in the state also have better legal rights than in many others, with a $15 minimum wage and guaranteed retirement benefits.

Janet Kim points to such programs as Hawaii's and Washington's as not only clear policy wins that could lead toward a new caring future, but also important moments where caregivers were empowered: "The campaigns in Hawaii and Washington mattered for us so much to show the power and momentum of people coming together," she says. "It's encouragement to keep on raising our voices and speaking truth to power, which can be hard even with our members. Caregiving is a very vulnerable issue, so there's a question of how you can feel your power when talking about something that can feel so personal and emotional."[16] Many caregivers, Kim says, feel like their struggle is a personal rather than a systemic failing, leading to shame and guilt—which can discourage activism. Organizing around caregiving can both help caregivers—or former caregivers, who may have more time and distance to engage in such work—to feel less alone, leading to policy change like the recent wins in Washington.

Such state-level policies provide possible models for national laws, but so too do initiatives already in place in other countries. A publication detailing care policies in countries belonging to the Organization for Economic Cooperation and Development[17] notes that twenty-two out of thirty-four of these nations mandated paid family leave for adult family members' health needs, with fifteen of those countries guaranteeing up to 80 percent wage replacement.[18] Belgium has a particularly long leave policy, offering up to twelve months of paid leave for caregivers, and the Scandinavian countries predictably offer the highest levels of pay replacement.[19] In 2014, Belgium also implemented official legal recognition for family caregivers, complete with a certificate renewed annually. This law was adopted with the intent of guaranteeing caregivers certain rights and allowing the government to offer more targeted support.[20]

Many other countries go beyond guaranteeing paid leave for caregivers. France and Sweden offer "caregiver credits," enabling family caregivers to earn public pension and retirement benefits even if they are unable to work.[21] Germany, Austria, and the Netherlands have so-called cash-for-care schemes, which vary in how they are implemented but can include direct payments to caregivers, home care respite, and other payments to support elderly and disabled citizens and their caregivers.[22] Ireland offers a Carer's Allowance to low-income caregivers who live with their care recipient and work fewer than fifteen hours per week outside the home.[23]

In Japan, well known as a rapidly aging country, the care crisis has already arrived. Although there's a strong cultural premium placed on caring for one's elders, there are simply not enough younger family members to do so. Japan had a shortage of 40,000 caregivers in 2015.[24] The nation has had to find new ways of managing care,[25] restructuring entire communities to accommodate elderly residents with dementia[26] and developing "care robots."[27] The country has also instituted a caregiving time bank.

Called Fureai Kippu ("caring relationship tickets"), it allows Japanese citizens to "bank" hours of service that they provide to elderly people in their community. (The hours are valued at higher rates for more demanding tasks, such as help with bathing.) The credits can then be transferred to their own elderly relatives who live elsewhere, or saved for their future use.[28] Fureai Kippu has operated since 1995 and has received considerable attention from currency theorists, as it represents a new form of electronic money—compassion as currency, as one article puts it[29]—but seems less well known beyond those circles. The recipients of care seem to prefer the system to care paid for in traditional money.[30]

THE NEXT BIG IDEAS

The United States could take a cue from any of these international models, though our current political climate makes the possibility seem distant. In our dissonant, polarized political landscape, any measure of humanity or communitarian interventions in problems like the scarcity of care gets shouted down by the right as socialism.

The long-standing American cultural premium on individualism and self-reliance (at least as an ideal, if not a reality) exacerbates the challenge. As Meghan O'Rourke, writing in *The Atlantic* during the coronavirus pandemic, points out, "We are so addicted to the concept of individual responsibility that we have a fragmented health-care system, a weak social safety net, and a culture of averting our eyes from other people's physical vulnerability."[31] The pandemic was a particularly stark reminder of the importance of societal interdependence. During the crisis, Americans were urged to help protect public health—especially those most vulnerable—by isolating ourselves, sacrificing work time and often income, and refraining from hoarding essential items such as hand sanitizer and (infamously) toilet paper. And yet Americans at large struggled with the idea of community-minded action; even measures as simple and beneficial as wearing masks in public became a depressingly contentious, partisan issue. Our systems were also stacked against it: many people were unable to take time off work, and our government, especially at the federal level, notably failed to provide leadership. American individualism has produced an enormous, structural failure to allow us to care for one another. Conservative political discourse frames our current system as one that encourages "choice"—language that, as studies show, decreases public support for more communitarian policies.[32] And, in turn, the lack of such policies constrains individuals' choices.

This vicious cycle has produced a fractured culture with a "screw you, buddy, I've got mine" ethos at its heart, but many activists and policymakers are trying to turn the tide. Although the federal landscape remains bleak, a growing movement of state and local policymakers and advocacy groups—such as Caring Across Generations and AARP—are pushing for changes across the United States, some incremental and some visionary. Incremental goals have included a push for a caregiver tax credit and paid leave for caregivers at the federal level. The proposed Family and Medical Insurance Leave (FAMILY) Act would create a national insurance fund, via paycheck and employer contributions, to provide partial wage replacement for those taking family medical or parental leave. Senator Kirsten Gillibrand (D-NY) first introduced the bill in 2013; in 2019, she and Representative Rosa DeLauro (D-CT) reintroduced the bill (HR 1185/S 463) in their respective chambers. The bill had not reached the floor of either body at the time of writing but the idea of paid leave was beginning to garner some Republican support.[33] Although the program, if enacted, would be less ambitious than the Universal Family Care plans discussed earlier, it would represent a huge improvement on current policy. Advocates, however, are not stopping with this idea: a coalition of progressive groups have launched a campaign called Paid Leave for All, which aims for a comprehensive federal paid leave policy by 2023.[34]

In July 2020, then presidential candidate Joe Biden added a major caregiving plank to his platform, calling for a $775 billion package investing in care for children, the elderly, and ill or disabled family members. The plan would include a $5,000 tax credit as well as Social Security credits for family caregivers; end Medicaid waitlists for home and community care; and add community health workers.[35] Biden, who was a single father when his sons were young, spoke to the economic pressures of all types of care—including those on paid caregivers—in announcing the proposals: "If we truly want to reward work in this country, we have to ease the financial burden of care that families are carrying. . . . We're trapped in a caregiving crisis, within an economic crisis within a health-care crisis."[36] As of this writing, it is unclear whether Biden's proposals will move forward or how they might dovetail with preexisting legislative initiatives, but the campaign's inclusion of caregiving as a major policy plank adds power to the growing chorus of voices calling for progress on issues around the subject.

Some advocates have also floated the idea of paying family caregivers directly for their labor via government programs, which at present mainly benefit caregivers indirectly. Although there's a long feminist history of demanding pay for various types of domestic and care labor—starting with scholar-activist Silvia Federici's 1975 book *Wages Against Housework* and continuing today with calls such as writer Kim Brooks's recent Mothers-Day-themed *New York Times* piece, "Forget Pancakes. Pay Mothers"[37]—actual policy traction, whether for homemakers or caregivers, has been negligible. Tax credits for caregivers can provide some financial relief, though they are far from direct pay. But one group of family caregivers does receive direct compensation: those caring for veterans. The Veterans Administration's Caregiver Support Program was initially available only to caregivers for recent veterans of Iraq and Afghanistan.[38] In 2018, however, Congress voted to expand to expand this program to pay family caregivers of vets of all wars.[39] For nonveterans needing care, however, support for caregivers is a patchwork of programs that can be difficult to access. In some states, such as California, Medicaid offers direct pay to low-income caregivers. In most states, Medicaid income-waiver programs allow individuals to receive care at home or in the community, even if the family has a higher income than the baseline threshold for Medicaid eligibility. Such programs vary by state.[40] That support is critical for middle-class families, since high-need care can quickly drain a family's resources, but demand for waiver programs is high and waiting lists can be punishingly long. According to "The Case for Inclusion"—an annual report assessing disability services nationwide, authored by staff from the nonprofit American Network of Community Options and Resources Foundation and United Cerebral Palsy—the number of people with intellectual and developmental disabilities on waiting lists for home and community-based services grew to 473,000 in 2020.[41]

Chris Gabbard—professor of English at the University of North Florida and the author of *A Life Beyond Reason*, a memoir of his late son August, who had cerebral palsy—relied on the Florida program's assistance.[42] Even with state assistance, it wasn't easy, he recounts: "It was really hard to get off the waiting list"—which, at the time of our conversation, had a thirteen-year wait. Gabbard and his wife, Ilene Chazan, finally appealed to their state senator for help.[43]

Despite the obstacles to access, the program made a crucial difference to Gabbard's family. After they were granted the waiver, Gabbard received direct pay in addition to support that enabled him to hire caregivers: "It became my second job. I was getting paid—not very much, something like $7 or $8 an hour, but it made a big difference," he says. "It stopped the hemorrhaging financially." Although caregiving deserves much more than minimum wage, Gabbard's story shows that even a modest compensation can make an immense difference to families.

Paying caregivers directly for their time is generally less costly than institutional or third-party care, and can be more comfortable for care recipients, who are able to stay at home and receive care from a familiar (and presumably loving) person. Such a measure could also help ameliorate the shortage of paid caregivers. But it would also represent a huge shift in cultural values, as Glenn points out in *Forced to Care*: "There lingers a sense of moral unease with paying family members to care for one another in some quarters," Glenn writes. "Critics of paid care argue that it is irresponsible to spend public funds on services that family members are supposed to provide for free and that compensation will undermine the sense of family obligation."[44] There are also concerns about the potential for elder abuse or neglect of care recipients, though these issues exist in any care relationship, paid or not.

An even bigger dream than direct pay for caregivers is something that would benefit all families: universal basic income. This concept received some traction in the 2020 Democratic presidential primary, specifically with candidate Andrew Yang, but is a long way from being a serious, viable policy proposal. Yang, who called the concept a Freedom Dividend, proposed a basic income—no strings attached—of $1,000 per month for every American adult.[45] In 2019, the high-poverty California city of Stockton (which I know well, as my grandparents lived there) piloted a small universal basic income program, providing $500 per month to 125 residents for eighteen months. One story from that program jumped out at me: a participant named Lorrine Parradela, stressed because her car had been totaled by another driver, was relieved to be able to get it fixed so she could support her mother, who had cancer and was at a hospital several hours away.[46] During the coronavirus pandemic, discussions of UBI returned to the forefront via conversations around stimulus payments to individuals. The ways that UBI could benefit strapped caregivers are legion but highly individual.

TOWARD CARING

Readers might be forgiven, at this point, for wondering how on earth the United States could go from a society with out-of-control, often profit-driven healthcare costs and essentially no provisions for supporting care to a humane, community-oriented society. I don't know, and I wish I did. What is clear to me is that we need not just a policy shift but a cultural shift on this issue—a change in attitudes to gendered labor, social ties, work, healthcare, family structures, and how we as a society fund the things we all collectively need. Rethinking care could be transformative for our society and could even be critical to the recovery of an economy battered by the coronavirus pandemic, as Gates Foundation cochair Melinda Gates argued in a 2020 *Washington Post* op-ed advocating for federally guaranteed paid family leave.[47] All we can do, as individuals, is to keep pushing for the changes we want to see.

Medium-scale solutions do exist. Caregiving consultancies, private care managers, and caregiving coaching services are starting to spring up—though these can be pricey. Caregiver Libby Brittain, who operated a care coaching service called Quilt, sought a more scalable solution and is starting a venture-backed software company to offer caregivers on-demand video classes and personal connections at a lower cost.[48] Informal care networks can be another solution, but they have to come together organically and usually on an ad hoc basis. Anne Boyer describes the "completely extralegal and unofficial" "inventive forms of love" that her friends devised to care for her while she was undergoing cancer treatment: "Some friends left, but some friends patchworked their money and time into care for me. The ones who had money wrote checks so that the ones with the capacity for thoughtful care could fly to me and help me empty the surgical drains stitched into my body. Some friends sent books, others sent mixtapes. Our solution to the problem of care is not scalable, was inadequate and provisional, but at least it got me through."[49]

Patchwork is an especially apt metaphor for care systems, referencing as it does that ultimate symbol for care and love: the quilt. Although informal networks currently tend to be a stopgap solution, formed by necessity, they have real promise as an intentionally chosen option for the future. As Boyer says, care networks like hers are not scalable, but the idea of expanding care to include groups of friends rather than a single caregiver is something individuals and families can adopt—and, at a societal level, a program like Japan's Fureai Kippu care bank could provide a broader model for a network approach. As we saw earlier in the book, care networks formed in the LGBTQ community in response to the AIDS crisis, and they continue today for needs of all kinds, from cancer to gender-confirmation surgery. Born of necessity and stigma, such care relationships have proved enriching and meaningful for both caregivers and their charges, as depicted in the recent documentary *5B*, which traces the history of nurses and volunteers caring for AIDS patients in 1980s San Francisco.

What makes networks of care an especially promising idea from my point of view is the ways they could reduce isolation and the heavy sense of personal responsibility that were so difficult for me through the hardest days of caregiving. Yet we're all busy and the strain of valuing independence runs deep: it was hard for me to imagine asking friends to take time off work to sit with Brad in the hospital or walk with him when he needed rehab. Instead, I leaned on my in-laws and paid for services where I could, asking friends mainly for dropped-off meals and other errands rather than hands-on help with the day-to-day. Although I don't think the solutions to the care crisis lie in caregivers doing more to help themselves, accepting and asking for more help can genuinely foster community and ease the load. Writer and activist Mia Birdsong offers an inspiring, broad vision for new, more caring social networks in her recent book *How We Show Up: Reclaiming Family, Friendship, and Community*. In it, she looks explicitly to the caring structures and networks of marginalized communities for "models of success and leadership that fundamentally value love, care, and generosity of resources and spirit."[50] If, taking a cue from Birdsong, we reject what she calls "toxic individualism" and the siloed constraints of keeping care within the conventional nuclear family, we can strive for, as she puts it, "connection, love, and care that is beyond the confines and the defaults and norms of . . . the dominant culture."[51] Although Birdsong's vision extends well beyond caregiving, it has obvious applications to the challenges of caring for one another.

When it comes to small-scale individual solutions, there are things that people who aren't (yet) caregivers can do to help family and friends who are. If this is you, and you're thinking of someone you know, offer specific help: recruit other friends to a care network and make and maintain the spreadsheet for it, set up a meal train, offer specific errands with a text like: "Hey, I'm going to Target, can I pick something up for you?" If your friend can't or won't accept hands-on help or attendance for the person they're caring for, offer to take their car for an oil change or pick up dry cleaning or take their kid to a movie. From far away, you can offer to make administrative calls, phone-tree needed information to others, or send care packages or a gift card for grocery delivery. Jumping into the fray to contribute, even if it feels awkward, helps to lessen the isolation of caregiving and build up the more community-minded, connected ethos we need if real changes in care are ever to come.

The coming wave of care needs may force a reckoning around caregiving, or it may simply make the burdens of more than 50 million Americans even heavier. Which will it be? Making the change that we all need and deserve won't be easy—not least because caregivers are mostly far too time-strapped to spend a lot of time on activism. If you don't even have time to see your doctor, how can you instigate a massive social upheaval that will overturn misogyny, reconcile Americans to social cooperation, and reframe the cultural meaning of care?

I don't have a single answer, but I wrote this book—in between kid carpools and my husband's eye surgeries and a lot of couples counseling and the days when I felt like I couldn't keep going, and sometimes at a hospital bedside and while we were worriedly sheltering in place during the coronavirus pandemic—to help to bring this ever more pressing issue into public view. It doesn't help anyone if thousands, or even millions, of us are all struggling alone in our isolated homes and hospital rooms and private moments of despair. We have to raise our voices, together, about how hard it is. Caregivers can't do right by the people we love and care for without recognition and help—we need acknowledgment for our work and the chance to live our lives. If society wants us to keep caring for others, it's going to have to show a little more care for us.

KEY SOURCES AND RESOURCES

This appendix offers an overview of 1) the most important works that helped me develop my thinking on caregiving and related issues, and 2) resources that may help the frayed caregivers among my readers. Although the notes contain complete attributions for the research included in this book, a listing of every single source I consulted would ultimately be less useful for readers than a shorter guide to key works—hence this narrative bibliography.

Several theoretical works especially informed my thinking around caregiving as a cultural phenomenon. Foremost among these was Evelyn Nakano Glenn's *Forced to Care: Coercion and Caregiving in America* (Cambridge, MA: Harvard University Press, 2010), an unflinching historical and sociological work that includes both family and paid forms of caregiving. Ai-jen Poo, with Ariane Conrad, wrote the thoughtful and thought-provoking *The Age of Dignity: Preparing for the Elder Boom in a Changing America* (New York: New Press, 2015), a crucial look at the growing importance of care in our society. Martha Nussbaum's *Creating Capabilities: The Human Development Approach* (Cambridge, MA: Belknap/Harvard University Press, 2011) offers an important grounding in the philosophy of care, while Susan Sontag's *Illness as Metaphor* (New York: Farrar, Straus & Giroux, 1977) remains an indispensable guide to thinking about sickness and suffering in Western culture.

A much more recent work, Ada Calhoun's *Why We Can't Sleep: Women's New Midlife Crisis* (New York: Grove Press, 2020), resonated deeply with me during my own Gen-X midlife crisis and, less personally, offers a critical synthesis of all the domestic inequality and care labor that drags women down. Calhoun's work is unusual among a recent spate of books treating similar issues in that it focuses heavily on caregiving for the ill and elderly. A number of the other recent books on gender and care are not directly germane to caregiving for the ill, but deeply informed my thinking. Many of these look at the nexus of parenting, domesticity, work, and feminism, among them Darcy Lockman's *All the Rage: Mothers, Fathers, and the Myth of Equal Partnership* (New York: Harper, 2019); Megan K. Stack's *Women's Work: A Reckoning with Work and Home* (New York: Doubleday, 2019); Gemma Hartley's *Fed Up: Emotional Labor, Women, and the Way Forward* (New York: HarperCollins, 2018); and Anne-Marie Slaughter's *Unfinished Business: Women, Men, Work, Family* (New York: Random House, 2015). All of these titles owe a debt, in my view, to the foundational works of Arlie Hochschild, whose *The Second Shift: Working Families and the Revolution at Home*, with Anne Machung (New York: Penguin, 1989; revised and updated edition, 2012), and, more recently, *The Managed Heart: Commercialization of Human Feeling* (Berkeley: University of California Press, 1983; updated edition, 2012) and *The Outsourced Self: What Happens When We Pay Others to Live Our Lives for Us* (New York: Picador, 2012) have been important sources for me as well. *The Outsourced Self* also offers a personal look at Hochschild's own work as a caregiver. For broad inspiration on rethinking our notions of family and how we provide care to one another, I recommend Mia Birdsong's recent *How We Show Up: Reclaiming Family, Friendship, and Community* (New York: Hachette, 2020).

A more economic slant on a related constellation of issues comes from Alissa Quart, in *Squeezed: Why Our Families Can't Afford America* (New York: Ecco, 2018). The *New York Times*'s March 9, 2020, investigation of the value of unpaid care labor, "Women's Unpaid Labor Is Worth $10,900,000," by Gus Wezerek and Kristen R. Ghodsee, provides a stark look at the economic implications of gendered (de)valuing of care. In general, the *New York Times* is providing very strong reporting on the rapidly changing landscape of care issues, particularly in the work of Claire Cain Miller. *The Atlantic* is also an invaluable source covering these issues. The landscape is likely to change even faster in the wake of coronavirus, and both outlets' coverage of the unfolding crisis was top-notch. I'd point to Helen Lewis's trenchant early article "The Coronavirus Is a Disaster for Feminism" in *The Atlantic* (March 19, 2020) as an exemplar.

Memoirs of caregiving—and memoirs of illness that also touch upon issues that relate to caregiving—abound. I found much to relate to and think about in Lorene Cary's *Ladysitting: My Year with Nana at the End of Her Century* (New York: W. W. Norton, 2019), about caring for her elderly grandmother; Abby Maslin's *Love You Hard: A Memoir of Marriage, Brain Injury, and Reinventing Love* (New York: Dutton, 2019), about her husband's traumatic brain injury; Arthur Kleinman's *The Soul of Care: The Moral Education of a Husband and a Doctor* (New York: Viking, 2019); and Glynnis MacNicol's *No One Tells You This: A Memoir* (New York: Simon & Schuster, 2018), as well as several essays in Briallen Hopper's *Hard to Love* (New York: Bloomsbury, 2019). Of the many memoirs of illness I've read, two that stand out for their perspectives on issues touching caregiving were Kate Bowler's *Everything Happens for a Reason: And Other Lies I've Loved* (New York: Random House, 2018) and Anne Boyer's lyrical memoir of breast cancer, *The Undying* (New York: Farrar, Straus & Giroux, 2019). Readers interested in historical caregiving may find interest in Louisa May Alcott's nursing memoir *Hospital Sketches* (Mineola, NY: Dover, 2006 [1863]), as well as the many fictional texts, such as *Middlemarch* and *Jane Eyre*, that I've engaged with in these pages.

How-to guides on caregiving are legion, and the gold standard of these is Gail Sheehy's *Passages in Caregiving: Turning Chaos into Confidence* (New York: William Morrow, 2010). Though Sheehy's advice on navigating emotional and relational pitfalls is excellent, the landscape on financial matters and healthcare policy has changed significantly since that time. For up-to-date advice, readers are best served by online resources.

The best, widest-ranging practical resource I know for caregivers is AARP's caregiving page: www.aarp.org/caregiving. Although to some extent its focus is on older adults, it covers topics ranging from finances to life balance, and it offers a deep bench of tools such as templates for living wills, guides for first-time caregivers, and care calculators. It's also actively maintained and responsive to current events that affect caregivers. In spring 2020, for instance, the page added a vast array of coronavirus content: how to boost loved ones' morale, navigating telehealth, identifying COVID-19-specific scams, and much, much more. I advise anyone who asks me where to start as a caregiver to go to the AARP site, regardless of age.

The Family Caregiver Alliance (www.caregiver.org) offers extensive resources and information for caregivers in a wide range of situations, as well as a wealth of statistics for researchers. The Caregiver Action Network (www.caregiveraction.org) houses many online resources as well as a unique (as far as I know) hotline specifically for caregivers, called the Caregiver Help Desk, which can be reached at 855-227-3640.

Another excellent resource is Caring Across Generations (caring across.org). As an advocacy organization, Caring Across Generations focuses on calls to action, but the site and their email lists for caregivers also offer such resources as practical assistance, tips, and news alerts concerning legislation or policies that may benefit caregivers.

For emotional support and connection I suggest starting with the Caregiver Space (www.thecaregiverspace.org), which runs numerous Facebook groups and offers resources helpfully organized by topic (burnout, grief, finances) and type of caregiver (e.g., for a parent, friend, or child). Many disease-specific organizations run support groups, either virtual or in-person, as do hospitals and cancer centers. Many disease advocacy groups can offer caregivers practical and financial support as well as social and emotional resources. (In my observation, dementia caregiving was relatively well supported in this regard.) If you have access to a hospital or medical-group social worker, ask them about specific local resources. I also strongly suggest searching online for local or state-level nonprofit groups that support caregivers. I had no idea until after the bulk of my caregiving days were done that there existed a statewide network of caregiver resource centers in California with state and grant funding, and that there is a local program near me. Sadly, it's all too easy for busy caregivers to miss such resources.

While not strictly dedicated to caregiving, *Burnout: The Secret to Unlocking the Stress Cycle* (New York: Ballantine Books, 2019), by Emily and Amelia Nagoski, offers an approach to stress management that I think can be of service to many caregivers. And for anyone who, like me, finds stress relief in cooking through a hard time, there's no better or warmer guide than Ella Risbridger's *Midnight Chicken (& Other Recipes Worth Living For)* (London: Bloomsbury, 2019), which touches on Risbridger's own life as a caregiver and cook.

· · ·

Because of the increasing and welcome visibility of caregiving—and especially in light of new developments related to COVID-19—the list of resources online is always growing. I maintain a list with links at my website, kawashington.com, where readers can also find a playlist for caregivers, links to my other writing, and information regarding my newsletter. If you have a suggestion for a resource that should be added to the list and/or a specific question for me, you can also contact me via the site. I'm always glad to hear from readers and grateful to learn from you.

ACKNOWLEDGMENTS

Writing this book has been a long-held dream—and a long path that I wasn't sure would ever actually lead anywhere. Some of the original drafts were scribbled by the side of my husband Brad Buchanan's bed in the Bone Marrow Transplant Unit on Davis 8. It has not been an easy journey for either of us—far less so for him. My first and biggest debt is to him. Brad, thank you for letting me tell this story, which is really yours, from my perspective. Thanks also to the nurses and physicians of the U.C. Davis Cancer Center and Davis 8—especially Melissa, Lori, Sara, and Dr. T, who saved Brad's life over and over when we thought hope was gone. A special thanks to Nancy Naitagaga and Emali Raseru, whose compassionate care for Brad was an incredible boon for our whole family.

Editors Sarah Blackwood and Sarah Mesle at *Avidly* gave my writing on caregiving its first home, with "Leslie's House of Nightmares." Megha Majumdar, my editor at *Catapult*, who fished my essay "Take You Me for a Sponge" out of the slush pile, took a chance on having me revise it, and was invaluable to helping me get my story out in the world. Portions of both essays and of another previously published work, "The Yoke of Duty: Of Caregiving and *Middlemarch*," which appeared in *Empty Mirror*, are included in this book in substantially altered form.

It has been a privilege to work with Beth Vesel, agent extraordinaire, who has been instrumental to this project's success. My editors at the *Sacramento Bee*, especially Tim Swanson and Jim Patrick, have provided invaluable encouragement and also patience when I blew deadlines for the sake of this project.

At Beacon Press, I thank my acquiring editor, Rakia Clark, for seeing promise in my proposal, and the rest of the team for supporting her in buying this book. My editor, Catherine Tung, has been instrumental in shaping and improving this story and shepherding me through to publication of my first book. Also at Beacon, my thanks go to managing editor Susan Lumenello and production director Marcy Barnes, copyeditor Steven Horne, proofreader Katie Blatt, and designer Louis Roe. It has been a pleasure to work with director of communications Pamela MacColl and with director of marketing Sanj Kharbanda, associate director of marketing Alyssa Hassan, and their respective teams; I am grateful for their enthusiasm for helping this book find its audience. Thanks also to audio operations assistant Isabel Tehan and audiobook reader Siiri Scott.

My writing mentor and dear friend Rae Gouirand held a space for my writing during the hardest times in Scribe Lab, at Tupelo, and with encouragement, texts, prophecy, and endless enthusiasm for my work. Molly Watson was a generous reader and dispenser of occasional tough love, emphasis on the love. Sarah Peterson, the friend who has been with me the longest, always, always asked how I was first. Jordanna Bailkin has been the best ex-roommate and cheerleader I've ever known. My tightest group of Extremely Online friends have provided endless love, memes, belief in me, and care packages of ice cream, not to mention advice on how to dip: Jana Lithgow, Meghan Kelly, Hannah Meehan, Jill Hermann-Wilmarth, Alexis Brett, Terri Coles, and Lisa Schmeiser. Thanks to my two fellow caregivers, Liz Kennish and Ella Risbridger, on different continents, who understood what it was like when nobody else did. Thanks to all of them, and many more friends than can be named, for getting me through the worst.

Support during crisis after crisis came from countless local friends, acquaintances, and even a few strangers who brought meals. Thanks especially to Ann Rolke for organizing the Meal Train, Scott and Kirsten Thurston for taking Lucy every Sunday, Amy Dixson for always welcoming Nora and providing adventures, Mary Huang for caring for the girls, Madeleine Lohman for those massages, and the generosity and support of the gym community at Aquila Fitness and my crew (not a metaphor) at River City Rowing Club.

To my in-laws Joe and Susan Buchanan, we could not have gotten through the hellish time that inspired this book without your steadfast support. Thank you for everything. James Buchanan, thank you for the stem cells. My dad Ernie Washington came to help, took the kids for weekends along with my always-kind stepmom Karen Washington, and bragged about me behind my back around my hometown. Thanks, Dad. The birth of my brother Peter Washington is my earliest memory, and I'm so glad he's always been there, through thick and thin and unending Scrabble games. Evalani Washington, I love you like the sister I never had. I wish my beloved grandparents Blair and Lois Erigero and my late mom Cathy Washington were here to see this book. It would not exist without their love and belief in me. And finally, to Nora and Lucy: my job may be writing, but my love for you goes beyond what I can express with words. You two are my greatest joy.

NOTES

INTRODUCTION: COLLATERAL DAMAGE

1. Evelyn Nakano Glenn, *Forced to Care: Coercion and Caregiving in America* (Berkeley: University of California Press, 2010), 35.

2. Arthur Kleinman, *The Soul of Care: The Moral Education of a Husband and a Doctor* (New York: Viking, 2019), 3.

3. Anne Boyer, *The Undying: Pain, Vulnerability, Mortality, Medicine, Art, Time, Dreams, Data, Exhaustion, Cancer, and Care* (New York: Farrar, Straus & Giroux, 2019), 30.

4. AARP Public Policy Institute and National Alliance for Caregiving, *Caregiving in the US: 2020 Report* (May 2020), 9, https://www.aarp.org/content/dam/aarp/ppi/2020/05/full-report-caregiving-in-the-united-states.doi.10.26419-2Fppi.00103.001.pdf. See also *Caregiving in the US: 2015 Report* (June 2015), 49, https://www.aarp.org/content/dam/aarp/ppi/2015/caregiving-in-the-united-states-2015-report-revised.pdf. Unless otherwise noted, subsequent references are to the 2015 report. .

5. The baby boom generation, by most estimates, includes those born between 1946 and 1964. In this book I use these dates and follow the Pew Research Center's other dates defining generations: Generation X includes those born 1965–1980 (born in 1972, I fall precisely in its middle); millennials are 1981–1996; and Generation Z is 1997–2012. See Michael Dimock, "Defining Generations: Where Millennials End and Generation Z Begins," Pew Research Center, January 17, 2019, https://www.pewresearch.org/fact-tank/2019/01/17/where-millennials-end-and-generation-z-begins.

6. The number of babies born in the US during those nineteen years is generally estimated at 76 million, though several million boomers have likely died since then. According to a 2014 estimate by the Population Reference Bureau, however, those deaths have been offset by population rise through immigration. See Kevin M. Pollard and Paola Scommegna, "Just How Many Baby Boomers Are There?" Population Reference Bureau, April 16, 2014, https://www.prb.org/justhowmanybabyboomersarethere.

7. Sabrina Tavernise, "U.S. Fertility Rate Fell to a Record Low, for Second Straight Year," *New York Times* (May 16, 2018), https://www.nytimes.com/2018/05/17/us/fertility-rate-decline-united-states.html.

8. Charles Hughes, "America's Fraying Social Ties," *Economics 21* (May 2017), https://economics21.org/html/america%E2%80%99s-fraying-social-ties-2360.html.

9. Aaron Carroll, "My Friend's Cancer Taught Me About a Hole in Our Health System," *New York Times*, March 25, 2019, https://www.nytimes.com/2019/03/25/upshot/my-friends-cancer-taught-me-about-a-hole-in-our-health-system.html.

10. AARP, "Family Caregiving," https://www.aarp.org/caregiving.

11. The year 2015 was the one with the most recently available statistics as of this writing. See *Caregiver Statistics: Demographics*, Family Caregiver Alliance, 2016, https://www.caregiver.org/caregiver-statistics-demographics.

12. Lynn Feinberg, personal interview with author, June 2018.

13. *Caregiver Statistics: Demographics*.

14. Boyer, *The Undying*, 51.

15. Kleinman, *The Soul of Care*, 3.

16. Emily Nagoski and Amelia Nagoski, *Burnout: The Secret to Unlocking the Stress* Cycle (New York: Ballantine Books, 2019), xii.

17. Kate Manne, *Down Girl: The Logic of Misogyny* (Oxford: Oxford University Press, 2018), 301.

18. Nagoski and Nagoski, xiv.

19. Manne, *Down Girl*, 301.

20. This ideal of woman as domestic paragon comes from a poem by the same name by now-obscure Victorian poet Coventry Patmore, originally published in 1854. The ideal the poem presents of a subservient wife who delights in caring for the home and fully inhabits the domestic sphere became a commonplace shorthand for Victorian gender stereotypes and has been widely invoked and criticized in the scholarly literature. Project Gutenberg edition: https://www.gutenberg.org/files/4099/4099-h/4099-h.htm.

21. My main focus here is on caring for sick adults, rather than the demands of caring for children who are ill—which often blur and overlap with parenting.

22. I consider the relationship between family caregiving and paid caregiving—specifically with reference to the economics of the two and my own need to hire paid caregivers—in more detail in chapter 5. For more on paid caregivers, see Glenn, *Forced to Care*, and Ai-Jen Poo, *The Age of Dignity: Preparing for the Elder Boom in a Changing America* (New York: New Press, 2015). A nonprofit advocacy group founded by Poo, Caring Across Generations, works on the explicit principle that family caregiver and paid caregiver rights are inextricably linked and a key social justice issue.

23. Caregiver Action Network, https://caregiveraction.org.

24. Although many long-term caregivers look after someone with chronic illness or disability, it's important to note that a large portion of the disabled community is fully independent and may rightly bristle at the notion that they might need a caregiver. However, some members of this community do need ongoing assistance. Disability awareness and activism is growing and overdue.

CHAPTER ONE: THE LEARNING CURVE

1. Ada Calhoun, *Why We Can't Sleep: Women's New Midlife Crisis* (New York: Grove Press, 2020), 8.

2. Calhoun, *Why We Can't Sleep*, 6.

3. Harper Lee, *To Kill a Mockingbird* (New York: J. B. Lippincott, 1960); see chapter 11.

4. E. O. Somerville and Martin Ross, *The Irish R.M.* (London: Sphere Books, 1985). The original book, a collection of humorous vignettes centering on a turn-of-the-century government official in rural Ireland, has also been turned into a television series.

5. Susan C. Reinhard, Carol Levine, and Sarah Samis, "Home Alone: Family Caregivers Providing Complex Chronic Care" (Washington, DC: AARP Public Policy Institute), 34.

6. Reinhard, Levine, and Samis, "Home Alone," 35.

7. Howard Gleckman, "Compassion Isn't Enough for Family Caregivers. They Need Training Too," *Forbes*, January 24, 2020, https://www.forbes.com/sites/howardgleckman/2020/01/14/compassion-isnt-enough-for-family-caregivers-they-need-training-too/amp.

8. Gleckman, "Compassion Isn't Enough."

9. Because donors tend to be a better match for people with similar genetic makeup, and there's a shortage of nonwhite and mixed-race donors, the registry is always especially looking for donors of color. For more information or to register as a potential donor, go to bethematch.org in the US.

CHAPTER TWO: THE THICK OF IT

1. Clostridium difficile—the full name—is an intestinal bacterium that causes severe diarrhea and is most common in hospital settings. It's named for the notorious difficulty of treating or eradicating it; it's also wildly contagious. Brad contracted it while he was at his most immune suppressed, as is common for stem cell transplant patients. Hospital protocols dictate various precautions for extremely transmissible conditions, mainly to avoid passing on infections to other patients via staff members.

2. Susan Sontag, *Illness as Metaphor* (New York: Farrar, Straus & Giroux, 1977), 6.

3. L. M. Montgomery, *Anne's House of Dreams* (New York: Bantam, 1981 [1922]).

4. *The Pool UK* has shut down and its archives are unfortunately no longer available online, but see also Ella Risbridger, *Midnight Chicken (& Other Recipes Worth Living For)* (London: Bloomsbury, 2019).

5. Montgomery, *Anne's House of Dreams*, 124–25.

6. Suzanne Edison, "When My Child Fell Ill," *Michigan Quarterly Review* 57:4 (Fall 2018): 544–45.

7. Kim Wyatt, "Terroir," *Michigan Quarterly Review* 57:4 (Fall 2018): 639–40.

8. Pronounced "two-lee," the word refers to a type of rush that thrives in Central Valley wetlands and also gave its name to a native variety of elk. Since many of California's marshy areas have been drained, it is less common.

9. The reasons why Brad got GvHD and others with sibling-matched donors don't aren't clear; stem cell transplants are still new enough that not everything about them is understood. When James and Brad were tested to see if James was a match to be a donor, they checked a number of proteins or markers, called HLA (human leukocyte antigen) markers, to see if they were a match. They look at ten markers; thirty-five years ago, when bone marrow transplants were brand-new, they had only four markers they could check for. It's now known that there are many other markers that medical science just doesn't have the technology to test for yet. What that all means is that there's no such thing as a guarantee of a perfect match, even though all ten of the markers they tested in Brad and James were a match. With a matched sibling-donor transplant, we were told, the chance of severe GvHD is somewhere around 10 percent.

10. Eliot depicts this cultural shift in medicine through the character of Lydgate, an ambitious doctor who wishes to found a new, professional, clean hospital. The hospital, however, is a charitable endeavor, one Dorothea Brooke supports with a large donation. In Lydgate's private practice he sees patients in their homes, where their relatives, friends, or hired help care for them. See George Eliot, *Middlemarch* (London: Penguin, 2015).

11. Abby Maslin, *Love You Hard* (New York: Dutton, 2019), 57.

12. Maslin, *Love You Hard*, 97.

CHAPTER THREE: ON HIS BLINDNESS

1. Charlotte Brontë, *Jane Eyre* (Oxford, UK: Oxford University Press, 1993), 469.

2. Brontë, *Jane Eyre*, 476.

3. John Milton, "Sonnet 19: When I Consider How My Light Is Spent," Poetry Foundation, https://www.poetryfoundation.org/poems/44750/sonnet-19-when-i-consider-how-my-light-is-spent.

4. Susan Silk and Barry Goldman, "How Not to Say the Wrong Thing," *Los Angeles Times*, April 7, 2013, https://www.latimes.com/opinion/op-ed/la-xpm-2013-apr-07-la-oe-0407-silk-ring-theory-20130407-story.html.

5. Montgomery, *Anne's House of Dreams*, 84.

6. Interestingly, in recent years Susan Gubar has become much more widely known for her *New York Times* column on living with cancer—which often touches on issues of caregiving—than for her academic work.

7. Sandra Gilbert and Susan Gubar, *The Madwoman in the Attic: The Woman Writer and the Nineteenth-Century Literary Imagination* (New Haven, CT: Yale University Press, 1979). For the classic fictional reimagining of—and sharp counterpoint to—*Jane Eyre*, see Jean Rhys's *Wide Sargasso Sea*, which retells the story from the point of view of the "mad wife" Bertha Mason, representing her as a victim of colonialism and prejudice.

8. Boyer, *The Undying*, 150.

9. Fox4 News Southwest Florida, "There's Now a Hotline Specifically for Caregivers," November 21, 2019, https://www.fox4now.com/news/national/theres-now-a-hotline-specifically-for-caregivers.

CHAPTER FOUR: CAREWORN

1. Ai-jen Poo, *The Age of Dignity*, 92.

2. The federal minimum wage as of 2020 is $7.25 per hour. State minimum wages are tracked by the Department of Labor at https://www.dol.gov/agencies/whd/minimum-wage/state.

3. Poo, *The Age of Dignity*, 90.

4. "Home Care Aides at a Glance," Facts 5, PHI, February 2014, 2, https://phinational.org/wp-content/uploads/legacy/phi-facts-5.pdf.

5. For a thorough (if dispiriting) overview of the legal history of paid care work in the US, see Glenn, *Forced to Care*, chapter 5.

6. AARP Public Policy Institute and National Alliance for Caregiving, *Caregiving in the US*, 49.

7. For more on the high costs of medical care, see chapter 6.

8. There are exceptions to this in some states, where Medicaid covers attendants, and in the case of some long-term care insurance, but the barriers to obtaining such care are high.

9. Barbara Ehrenreich, *Bright-Sided: How the Relentless Promotion of Positive Thinking Has Undermined America* (New York: Metropolitan Books, 2009).

10. Kate Bowler, *Everything Happens for a Reason: And Other Lies I've Loved* (New York: Random House, 2018), 112–13.

11. Bowler, *Everything Happens*, 118.

12. Helen Lewis, "The Coronavirus Is a Disaster for Feminism," *Atlantic*, March 19, 2020, https://www.theatlantic.com/international/archive/2020/03/feminism-womens-rights-coronavirus-covid19/608302.

13. Zoe Fenson, "It's So Much More Than Cooking," *Week*, October 2, 2019, https://theweek.com/articles/864481/much-more-than-cooking.

14. Megan K. Stack, *Women's Work: A Reckoning with Work and Home* (New York: Doubleday, 2019), 327.

CHAPTER FIVE: TO A CRISP

1. Unless otherwise noted, figures and statistics in this section are derived from the publication *Caregiver Statistics: Demographics*, by the Family Caregiver Alliance, 2016, https://www.caregiver.org/caregiver-statistics-demographics.

2. Calhoun, *Why We Can't Sleep*, 83.

3. Ninety-six percent of family caregivers assist with ADLs (activities of daily living); see *Caregiver Statistics: Demographics.*

4. M. Glantz et al., "Gender Disparity in the Rate of Partner Abandonment in Patients with Serious Medical Illness," *Cancer* 115:22 (November 2009), https://www.ncbi.nlm.nih.gov/pubmed/19645027.

5. Calhoun, *Why We Can't Sleep*, 128–29.

6. Jennifer Liu, "Your Happiness Is More Likely to Hit Rock Bottom at 47.2—but There's an Upside, Says New Research," CNBC, January 16, 2020, https://www.cnbc.com/2020/01/16/happiness-hits-rock-bottom-at-age-47-2-according-to-new-research.html.

7. Calhoun, *Why We Can't Sleep*, 82.

8. *Caregiver Profile: The Millennial Caregiver* (Bethesda, MD: National Alliance for Caregiving and AARP Public Policy Institute, August 2015), https://

www.caregiving.org/wp-content/uploads/2015/05/Caregiving-in-the-US-2015_-Millennial_CG-Profile-FINAL.pdf.

9. "LGBT Caregivers," National LGBT Cancer Network, https://cancer-network.org/cancer-information/lgbt-caregivers, accessed August 19, 2020.

10. Anna Muraco and Karen Fredriksen-Goldsen, "That's What Friends Do: Informal Caregiving for Chronically Ill Midlife and Older Lesbian, Gay, and Bisexual Adults," *Journal of Social and Personal Relationships* (March 2011), https://journals.sagepub.com/doi/abs/10.1177/0265407511402419.

11. *Caregiver Statistics: Demographics*.

12. "LGBT Caregivers."

13. Rebecca Makkai, *The Great Believers* (New York: Viking, 2018).

14. Tori Truscheit, "When You're Trans, Living with Your Parents Can Be Complicated," *BuzzFeed*, July 1, 2019, https://www.buzzfeednews.com/article/toritruscheit/young-transgender-millennials-living-at-home-homelessness.

15. Note: The original source denotes this ethnic group by use of the term "Hispanic" (specifying that this category does not include those of African American or white descent), which many in the community now consider dated. Throughout this book, I use the term "Latinx" in preference to Hispanic.

16. I know of no demographic guides that break out statistics for Native American or other, smaller marginalized groups.

17. Aisha Adkins, "As a Millennial Caregiver, Here's How Universal Family Care Could Make My Sacrifice Easier," *Blavity*, March 2, 2020, https://blavity.com/as-a-millennial-caregiver-heres-how-universal-family-care-could-make-my-sacrifice-easier?category1=opinion.

18. *Caregiver Statistics: Demographics*.

19. Glenn, *Forced to Care*, 2.

20. Anne-Marie Slaughter, *Unfinished Business: Women, Men, Work, Family* (New York: Random House, 2015), 94–95.

21. Slaughter, *Unfinished Business*, 96.

22. Glenn, *Forced to Care*, 5.

23. Gwendolyn Brooks, "Jessie Mitchell's Mother," from *Selected Poems* (New York: Harper & Row, 1963). Reprinted at https://www.poetryfoundation.org/poems/43316/jessie-mitchells-mother.

24. *Caregiver Statistics: Demographics*.

25. Karen Clayton, *Demystifying Hospice: Inside the Stories of Patients and Their Caregivers* (Lanham, MD: Rowman and Littlefield, 2018), 6.

26. Glenn, *Forced to Care*, 5.

27. Boyer, *The Undying*, 54–55.

28. *Caregiver Statistics: Demographics*.

29. *Caregiver Statistics: Demographics*.

30. "In recent years, the role of family caregivers has greatly expanded from coordinating and providing personal care and household chores to include medical or nursing tasks (such as wound care and administering injections). These difficult nursing tasks were provided in hospitals and nursing homes and by home care providers, but increasingly, family members are called on to perform these tasks with little training or professional support." See Donald Redfoot, Lynn Feinberg, and Ari Houser, "The Aging of the Baby Boom and

the Growing Care Gap: A Look at Future Declines in the Availability of Family Caregivers," AARP Public Policy Institute, *Insight on the Issues* 85 (August 2013): 2.

31. Redfoot, Feinberg, and Houser, "The Aging of the Baby Boom," 1.

32. Tracy Grant, "I Was My Husband's Caregiver as He Was Dying of Cancer. It Was the Best Seven Months of My Life," *Washington Post*, August 30, 2016, https://www.washingtonpost.com/news/inspired-life/wp/2016/08/30/i-was-my-husbands-caregiver-as-he-was-dying-of-cancer-it-was-the-best-seven-months-of-my-life.

33. The long history of maltreatment of disabled people is far too big a subject for the scope of this book. The field of disability studies has expanded rapidly in recent years; a good introductory resource is UCLA's Disability Studies guide online: https://guides.library.ucla.edu/disability-studies/books.

34. Sara Luterman, "There Is Nothing Loving About Killing Disabled People," *Washington Post*, January 1, 2020, https://www.washingtonpost.com/outlook/2020/01/01/there-is-nothing-loving-about-killing-disabled-people.

35. Julie Gregory, *Sickened: The Memoir of a Munchausen by Proxy Childhood* (New York: Bantam, 2003).

36. "How to Reclaim Your Life: Five Tips to Break Out of Isolation," CaregiverStress.com, https://www.caregiverstress.com/senior-activities/social-issues/how-to-reclaim-your-life-5-tips-to-break-out-of-isolation.

37. Paula Span, "Caregiving Is Hard Enough. Isolation Can Make It Unbearable," *New York Times*, August 4, 2017, https://www.nytimes.com/2017/08/04/health/caregiving-alzheimers-isolation.html.

38. *Caregiver Statistics: Demographics.*

39. Span, "Caregiving Is Hard Enough."

40. Briallen Hopper, *Hard to Love* (New York: Bloomsbury, 2019), 221.

41. Hopper, *Hard to Love*, 226–27.

42. Janet Kim, personal communication with author, October 2019.

43. Nagoski and Nagoski, *Burnout*.

CHAPTER SIX: INVALUABLE

1. *Friday Night Lights* is interesting for its many depictions of caregiving as well, especially the first season's in-depth look at the burden on sophomore quarterback Matt Saracen caring for his grandmother, who has dementia, while his father serves in Iraq.

2. Brad Buchanan, *The Scars, Aligned* (Georgetown, KY: Finishing Line Press, 2019).

3. Eliot, *Middlemarch*, 450.

4. Eliot, *Middlemarch*, 453.

5. Glenn, *Forced to Care*, 3.

6. Rachel Khong, *Goodbye, Vitamin* (New York: Picador, 2017).

7. Viet Thanh Nguyen, "I'd Love You to Want Me," in *The Refugees* (New York: Grove Press, 2017), 108.

8. Louisa May Alcott, *Little Women* (New York: Grosset & Dunlap, 1947 [1978 printing; originally published 1868]), 178–79.

9. Cited in Poo, *The Age of Dignity*, 64.

10. Gail Sheehy, *Passages in Caregiving: Turning Chaos into Confidence* (New York: William Morrow, 2010), 49.

11. Chabeli Carranza, "America's First Female Recession," *The 19th*, August 2, 2020, https://19thnews.org/2020/08/americas-first-female-recession.

12. Chuck Rainville, Laura Skufca, and Laura Mehegan, *Family Caregiving and Out-of-Pocket Costs: 2016 Report* (Washington, DC: AARP Research, November 2016), https://doi.org/10.26419/res.00138.001. See also Jo Ann Jenkins, "Caregiving Costly to Family Caregivers," AARP online, November 14, 2016, https://www.aarp.org/caregiving/financial-legal/info-2017/family-caregiving-costly-jj.html.

13. Kristina Brown, "My Family Faces an Impossible Choice: Caring for Our Mom, or Building Our Future," *Washington Post*, October 31, 2019, https://www.washingtonpost.com/outlook/my-family-faces-an-impossible-choice-caring-for-our-mom-or-building-our-future/2019/10/31/755526ea-f9c6-11e9-8906-ab6b60de9124_story.html; Deborah Bonello, "The Unequal Financial Burden for Black Caregivers," *Ozy*, January 16, 2020, https://www.ozy.com/news-and-politics/the-particular-burden-of-caregiving-on-black-families/256471.

14. Cited in Glenn, *Forced to Care*, 3.

15. Cited in Calhoun, *Why We Can't Sleep*, 82.

16. Eduardo Porter, "Why Aren't More Women Working? They're Caring for Parents," *New York Times*, August 29, 2019, https://www.nytimes.com/2019/08/29/business/economy/labor-family-care.html.

17. Slaughter, *Unfinished Business*, 87.

18. Gus Wezerek and Kristen R. Ghodsee, "Women's Unpaid Labor Is Worth $10,900,000," *New York Times*, March 9, 2020, https://www.nytimes.com/interactive/2020/03/04/opinion/women-unpaid-labor.html.

19. Wezerek and Ghodsee, "Women's Unpaid Labor Is Worth $10,900,000."

20. Slaughter, *Unfinished Business*, 54.

21. A lively debate has arisen about that term, originally coined in 1983 by sociologist Arlie Hochschild in *The Managed Heart: Commercialization of Human Feeling* (Berkeley: University of California Press, 2012 [updated edition]), to describe the commodification of affect in the workplace by such workers as flight attendants. For them, being pleasant no matter how they feel internally is a critical part of the job, and Hochschild originally meant the term to apply only to paid work—but to describe the internal contradictions and pain of managing one's emotions for pay—as she makes clear in an interview with journalist Julie Beck in "The Concept Creep of Emotional Labor," *Atlantic*, November 26, 2018, https://www.theatlantic.com/family/archive/2018/11/arlie-hochschild-housework-isnt-emotional-labor/576637. That "concept creep" around emotional labor stems in no small part from the recent work of Gemma Hartley, whose viral *Harper's Bazaar* article and subsequent book use the term to mean everything from picking up your kid's socks to arranging your mother-in-law's funeral. See Annaliese Griffin, "The Definition of Emotional Labor Has Changed. Don't Fight It," *Quartzy*, January 20, 2019, https://qz.com/quartzy/1522945/the-definition-of-emotional-labor-has-changed-dont-fight-it/;

Gemma Hartley, "Women' Aren't Nags—We're Just Fed Up," *Harper's Bazaar*, September 27, 2017, https://www.harpersbazaar.com/culture/features/a12063822/emotional-labor-gender-equality/; and Gemma Hartley, *Fed Up: Emotional Labor, Women, and the Way Forward* (New York: Harper Collins, 2018).

22. Arlie Hochschild with Anne Machung, *The Second Shift: Working Families and the Revolution at Home* (revised ed., New York: Penguin, 2012), 269.

23. Christina Ianzito, "Family Caregiving Worth $470 Billion a Year, AARP Finds," *AARP Blog: Take Care*, July 16, 2015, https://blog.aarp.org/2015/07/16/family-caregiving-worth-470-billion-a-year-aarp-finds.

24. Sheehy, *Passages in Caregiving*, 48.

25. Feinberg, interview with the author, June 2018.

26. US Department of Labor Wage and Hour Division, "Families First Coronavirus Response Act: Employer Expanded Family and Medical Leave Requirements," https://www.dol.gov/agencies/whd/pandemic/ffcra-employer-paid-leave.

27. Joan C. Williams, "Real Life Horror Stories from the World of Pandemic Motherhood," *New York Times*, August 6, 2020, https://www.nytimes.com/2020/08/06/opinion/mothers-discrimination-coronavirus.html.

28. Samantha Young, "States Seek Relief for Family Caregivers," *New York Times*, March 20, 2019, https://www.nytimes.com/2019/03/20/well/family/states-seek-financial-relief-for-family-caregivers.html.

29. National Health Expenditure Data, Centers for Medicare and Medicaid Services, https://www.cms.gov/Research-Statistics-Data-and-Systems/Statistics-Trends-and-Reports/NationalHealthExpendData/NationalHealthAccountsHistorical.

30. Personal correspondence, 2016. See also Kate Washington, "What Cancer Can Cost (Even with Insurance)," *Billfold*, February 6, 2017, https://www.thebillfold.com/2017/02/what-cancer-can-cost-even-with-insurance.

31. See Bruce Fagel, "Medical Malpractice Damages after the Cuevas Case," *Plaintiff Magazine*, June 2017, https://www.plaintiffmagazine.com/recent-issues/item/medical-malpractice-damages-after-the-case-cuevas-case-case, and "Personal Injury Claims Dealt Another Blow by California Court," *FindLaw* online, https://practice.findlaw.com/practice-guide/personal-injury-claims-dealt-another-blow-by-california-court.html.

32. See Wezerek and Ghodsee, "Women's Unpaid Labor Is Worth $10,900,000."

33. Glenn, *Forced to Care*, 16.

34. Glenn, *Forced to Care*, 18.

35. Glenn, *Forced to Care*, 35.

36. Glenn, *Forced to Care*, 24.

37. Louisa May Alcott, *Hospital Sketches* (Mineola, NY: Dover, 2006 [1863]), 20.

38. Poo, *The Age of Dignity*, 99.

39. Calomel was mercury chloride, a dangerous purgative used as a medicine at the time. Glenn, *Forced to Care*, 27 and 39–40.

40. Poo, *The Age of Dignity*, 99.

41. Alissa Quart, *Squeezed: Why Our Families Can't Afford America* (New York: Ecco, 2018), 77. *Squeezed* touches only lightly on caregiving but is a trenchant exploration of how rising basic costs (especially of childcare and housing), stagnant wages, and the increasing precarity of work make middle-class life unaffordable for millions of Americans.

42. Poo, *The Age of Dignity*, 8.

43. Glenn, *Forced to Care*, 41.

44. Quart, *Squeezed*, 77.

45. Martha Nussbaum, *Creating Capabilities: The Human Development Approach* (Cambridge, MA: Harvard University Press, 2011).

46. Nussbaum, *Creating Capabilities*, 151–52.

47. Darcy Lockman, *All the Rage: Mothers, Fathers, and the Myth of Equal Partnership* (New York: Harper, 2019), 258.

48. Poo, *The Age of Dignity*, 69.

49. Slaughter, *Unfinished Business*, 57.

CHAPTER SEVEN: A LACK OF REASONABLE OPTIONS

1. AARP Public Policy Institute and National Alliance for Caregiving, *Caregiving in the US*, 77.

2. Calhoun, *Why We Can't Sleep*, 68.

3. AARP Public Policy Institute and National Alliance for Caregiving, *Caregiving in the US*, 76.

4. Laura Richards, "Caught in the Middle: Caring for Your Kids and Your Aging Parents," *Healthline: Parenthood*, https://www.healthline.com/health/parenting/caring-for-your-babies-and-your-aging-parents.

5. Lorene Cary, *Ladysitting: My Year with Nana at the End of Her Century* (New York: Norton, 2019).

6. Allison Pearson, *How Hard Can It Be?* (New York: St. Martin's Press, 2018), 315.

7. Pearson, *How Hard Can It Be?*, 320.

8. Lockman, *All the Rage*, 258.

9. Poo, *The Age of Dignity*, 30.

10. Poo, *The Age of Dignity*, 30.

11. In 2015, the median income was $37,700 for Black caregivers and $38,600 for Latinx versus $62,200 for whites and $74,700 for Asian Americans. See *Caregiving in the US*, 76.

12. Rohinton Mistry, *Family Matters* (New York: Knopf, 2002), 206.

13. Alice Walker, *The Color Purple* (New York: Harcourt, 1982), 46.

14. Walker, *The Color Purple*, 53.

15. Walker, *The Color Purple*, 87.

16. Hopper, *Hard to Love*, 228.

17. David Allen and Abhay Vasavada, "Cataract and Surgery for Cataract," *British Medical Journal* 333:7559 (July 15, 2006), https://www.ncbi.nlm.nih.gov/pmc/articles/PMC1502210.

18. Mira T. Lee, *Everything Here Is Beautiful* (New York: Viking, 2018), 310–11.

19. Gabrielle Burton, *Searching for Tamsen Donner* (Omaha: University of Nebraska Press, 2009), 12. See also Gabrielle Burton, *Impatient with Desire* (New York: Hyperion, 2010).

20. Rituxan is not technically a chemotherapy drug but instead an antibody therapy.

21. Cary, *Ladysitting*, 216.

22. Cary, *Ladysitting*, 221.

23. Poo, *The Age of Dignity*, 127.

24. Rose M. Rubin and Shelley I. White-Means, "Informal Caregiving: Dilemmas of Sandwiched Caregivers," *Journal of Family and Economic Issues* 30:3 (September 2009), https://link.springer.com/article/10.1007/s10834-009-9155-x.

25. See Sarah Boyle, "Remembering the Origins of the Self-Care Movement," *Bust*, https://bust.com/feminism/194895-history-of-self-care-movement.html.

26. Evette Dionne, "For Black Women, Self-Care Is a Radical Act," *Ravishly*, March 9, 2015, https://ravishly.com/2015/03/06/radical-act-self-care-black-women-feminism.

27. Shanesha Brooks-Tatum, "Subversive Self-Care: Centering Black Women's Wellness," Feminist Wire, November 9, 2012, https://thefeministwire.com/2012/11/subversive-self-care-centering-black-womens-wellness.

CHAPTER EIGHT: SOMETHING IS NOT RIGHT

1. Survivors of cancer and other severe illness, for instance, are known to be at risk for PTSD, as described by Sophia Smith in "Cancer and PTSD: What You Need to Know," Young Survival Coalition, https://blog.youngsurvival.org/cancer-and-ptsd-what-you-need-to-know.

2. See "PTSD: National Center for PTSD," US Department of Veterans Affairs, https://www.ptsd.va.gov.

3. "Posttraumatic Stress Disorder," fact sheet, American Psychiatric Association, DSM-5 Collection. Available at https://www.psychiatry.org/psychiatrists/practice/dsm/educational-resources/dsm-5-fact-sheets.

4. Smith, "Cancer and PTSD: What You Need to Know."

5. "DSM-5 Criteria for PTSD," Brainline, February 22, 2018, https://www.brainline.org/article/dsm-5-criteria-ptsd.

6. James Bender, "What Are the Differences Between PTS and PTSD?," Brainline, December 9, 2013, https://www.brainline.org/article/what-are-differences-between-pts-and-ptsd.

7. Ella Risbridger, "Don't Let Us Get Sick: A Study of the Plague Years," March 15, 2020, https://ella.substack.com/p/dont-let-us-get-sick-478.

8. E. Azoulay et al., "Risk of Post-Traumatic Stress Symptoms in Family Members of Intensive Care Unit Patients," *American Journal of Respiratory Critical Care Medicine* (May 1, 2005), https://www.ncbi.nlm.nih.gov/pubmed/15665319.

9. Zora Neale Hurston, *Their Eyes Were Watching God* (New York: Harper & Row, 1990), 183.

10. Jennifer McAdam, et al., "Psychological Symptoms of Family Members of High-Risk Intensive Care Unit Patients," *American Journal of Critical Care* 21:6 (November 2012), http://ajcc.aacnjournals.org/content/21/6/386.full.pdf.

11. For a short overview of vicarious trauma, particularly linked to counseling professionals, see Fact Sheet #9, "Vicarious Trauma," issued by the American Counseling Association: https://www.counseling.org/docs/trauma-disaster/fact-sheet-9---vicarious-trauma.pdf.

12. Fact Sheet #9.

13. Judith Graham, "For Some Caregivers, the Trauma Lingers," *New York Times*, January 30, 2013, https://newoldage.blogs.nytimes.com/2013/01/30/for-some-caregivers-the-trauma-lingers.

14. Jennifer Levin, "I Was My Dad's Caregiver Through His Fatal Illness. I Had No Idea I'd Be at Risk for PTSD," *Washington Post*, Wellness, December 12, 2018, https://www.washingtonpost.com/lifestyle/wellness/i-was-my-dads-caregiver-through-his-fatal-illness-i-had-no-idea-id-be-at-risk-for-ptsd/2018/12/10/1f8df508-f4e4-11e8-aeea-b85fd44449f5_story.html.

15. Ludwig Bemelmans, *Madeline* (New York: Puffin, 2000 [1939]).

16. Glynnis MacNicol, *No One Tells You This* (New York: Simon & Schuster, 2018), 150.

17. Makkai's novel focuses in part on a straight woman as caregiver, and Makkai is herself straight; as such, the novel has been subject to criticism. *The Great Believers* depicts the complex networks of caregiving among the men in the (fictional) gay community it explores, but it largely leaves out the vital role of the lesbian community in both caring for and engaging in activism with the victims of AIDS. See Kira Brekke, "How Lesbians' Role in the AIDS Crisis Helped Bring Gay Men and Women Together," *Huffington Post*, October 9, 2015, https://tinyurl.com/y46qqexp. For more on the role of lesbians, see the oral history by Zaahira Wyne, "The Women Who Fought AIDS: 'It Was Never Not Our Battle,'" *Vice*, August 28, 2015, https://www.vice.com/en_us/article/mbqjqp/the-women-who-fought-aids-it-was-never-not-our-battle; the documentary *Quiet Heroes*, which looks at lesbian medical professionals who treated AIDS patients in Salt Lake City, discussed in John Paul Brammer's piece "Meet the 'Quiet Heroes' Who Cared for AIDS Patients in the '80s," *Them*, August 23, 2018, https://www.them.us/story/quiet-heroes-doc; and more.

18. Dan Lopez, "A Burdensome Memory: Rebecca Makkai's *The Great Believers*," *Los Angeles Review of Books*, August 4, 2018, https://lareviewofbooks.org/article/a-burdensome-memory-rebecca-makkais-the-great-believers/#!.

19. Makkai, *The Great Believers*, 360.

20. Makkai, *The Great Believers*, 407.

21. Makkai, *The Great Believers*, 405.

CHAPTER NINE: THE AFTERMATH

1. Sarah Stankorb, "Isolation and 'Impossible Choices': When Caregiving Goes into Lockdown," *Lily*, April 8, 2020, https://www.thelily.com/isolation-and-impossible-choices-when-caregiving-goes-into-lockdown.

2. Kleinman, *The Soul of Care*, 3.

3. We get few details on this surgery—and since the story takes place circa 1900 it seems far-fetched—but Gilbert conceives of the idea while examining carbuncles (large boils) on Dick's neck. The mention of the carbuncles subtly underscores the difficulty Leslie must have in caring for Dick; carbuncles could easily become infected, one more thing for her to tend to.

4. Montgomery, *Anne's House of Dreams*, 183.

5. Montgomery, *Anne's House of Dreams*, 184. Brad's story, like George and Dick Moore's, has a bizarre genetic twist. He has changed on a genetic level, though it's not apparent to the eye. He is a chimera now—in scientific terms, an organism with two different genetic signatures. In the stem cell transplant, all of the cells of his immune system were wiped out through intensive chemo and radiation, and stem cells from his brother's blood repopulated his marrow. Occasionally, natural chimerism results in two differently colored eyes, so the fictional George and Dick Moore may have been chimeras of a different sort.

6. Montgomery, *Anne's House of Dreams*, 209.

7. "Beginning Again After Caregiving Ends, a Six-Week Course," Care-Giving.com, https://www.caregiving.com/courses/beginning-again-after-caregiving-ends-a-6-week-course.

8. Donna Schempp, "When Caregiving Ends," Family Caregiver Alliance (2013), https://www.caregiver.org/when-caregiving-ends.

9. Mary Helen Berg, "What Happens When Caregiving Ends," *AARP Bulletin*, November 6, 2018, https://www.aarp.org/caregiving/life-balance/info-2018/after-caregiving-ends.html.

10. MacNicol, *No One Tells You This*.

11. MacNicol, *No One Tells You This*, 235–36.

12. MacNicol, *No One Tells You This*, 236.

13. Alcott, *Little Women*, 480.

14. MacNicol, *No One Tells You This*, 286.

15. MacNicol, *No One Tells You This*, 287.

16. Mary Beth Keane, *Ask Again, Yes* (New York: Scribner, 2019), 165–66.

CONCLUSION: DAMAGE CONTROL

1. Janet Kim, personal communication with author, October 2019.

2. "Universal Family Care," website, https://universalfamilycare.org.

3. Benjamin W. Veghte, Alexandra L. Bradley, Marc Cohen, and Heidi Hartmann, eds. *Designing Universal Family Care: State-Based Social Insurance Programs for Early Child Care and Education, Paid Family and Medical Leave, and Long-Term Services and Supports* (Washington, DC: National Academy of Social Insurance, 2019), https://universalfamilycare.org/wp-content/uploads/2019/06/Designing-Universal-Family-Care_Digital-Version_FINAL.pdf.

4. Jenna Gerry, personal conversation with author, October 2019.

5. Adkins, "As a Millennial Caregiver, Here's How Universal Family Care Could Make My Sacrifice Easier."

6. "Family and Medical Leave Act," US Department of Labor website, https://www.dol.gov/whd/fmla.

7. Boyer, *The Undying*, 29.

8. Janet Kim, personal communication with author, October 2019. Oregon's statute was enacted in October 2019 and goes into effect in 2023. See also Veghte, Bradley, Cohen, and Hartmann, *Designing Universal Family Care*.

9. "Caregiving + My Job," Legal Aid at Work, fact sheet, https://legalaidatwork.org/wp-content/uploads/2016/12/Cancer-My-Job-Updated-3.2018-00530215.pdf.

10. Sharon Terman, personal conversation with author, October 2019.

11. §1908a, Vermont Partnership for Long-Term Care (November 2018), Title 33, Human Services Vermont Statutes Online, https://legislature.vermont.gov/statutes/section/33/019/01908a.

12. "Family Caregivers Win in Hawai'i!" Caring Across Generations website, July 7, 2017, https://caringacross.org/family-caregivers-win-hawaii.

13. Rachel M. Cohen, "Washington Becomes First State to Approve Publicly Funded Long-Term Care," *Intercept*, April 26, 2019, https://theintercept.com/2019/04/26/washington-state-long-term-care.

14. Bryce Covert, "Washington State Has Created the Nation's First Social-Insurance Program for Long-Term Care," *Nation*, May 13, 2019, https://www.thenation.com/article/long-term-care-insurance-washington-elderly.

15. Poo, *The Age of Dignity*, 149.

16. Kim, personal conversation with author, October 2019.

17. Founded in 1961, the OECD has thirty-four member countries, all of which have relatively high-income economies, among them the US, Canada, most of the Western European nations, Japan, Turkey, Australia, Chile, and Mexico.

18. The rates of both wage-replacement and leave guarantees are slightly higher for parental leaves and children's health needs. WORLD Policy Analysis Center, "Paid Leave for Family Illness: A Detailed Look Across OECD Countries" (2018), https://www.worldpolicycenter.org/sites/default/files/WORLD%20Report%20-%20Family%20Medical%20Leave%20OECD%20Country%20Approaches_0.pdf.

19. OECD, "Policies to Support Family Carers," 122, https://www.oecd.org/els/health-systems/47884889.pdf.

20. Meredith Hughes, "International Approaches to Family Caregiving: Lessons for the United States," master's thesis (University of Pittsburgh, 2017), http://d-scholarship.pitt.edu/31119.

21. John Jankowski, "Caregiver Credits in France, Germany, and Sweden: Lessons for the United States," *Social Security Bulletin* 71: 4 (2011), https://www.ssa.gov/policy/docs/ssb/v71n4/v71n4p61.html.

22. Barbara Da Roit and Blanche Le Bihan, "Similar and Yet So Different: Cash-for-Care in Six European Countries' Long-Term Care Policies," *Millbank Quarterly* 88:3 (September 2010), https://www.ncbi.nlm.nih.gov/pmc/articles/PMC3000929.

23. Citizen Information Ireland, "Carer's Allowance," https://www.citizensinformation.ie/en/social_welfare/social_welfare_payments/carers/carers_allowance.html.

24. "Ageing and Innovation in Japan: Fact Sheet," Global Coalition on Aging and Health and Global Policy Institute, https://globalcoalitiononaging.com/wp-content/uploads/2018/12/ENG-Fact-Sheet.pdf.

25. T. R. Reid, "Aging in Japan: Free Glasses, Extra 'Walk' Time, Elder Love Stories," *AARP Bulletin*, May 17, 2018, https://www.aarp.org/health/healthy-living/info-2018/japan-elderly-aging-society.html

26. Justin McCurry, "'Dementia Towns': How Japan Is Evolving for Its Ageing Population," *Guardian*, January 14, 2018, https://www.theguardian.com/world/2018/jan/15/dementia-towns-japan-ageing-population.

27. "Japan Is Embracing Nursing-Care Robots," *Economist*, November 23, 2017, https://www.economist.com/business/2017/11/23/japan-is-embracing-nursing-care-robots.

28. Poo, *The Age of Dignity*, 135–36.

29. "Fureai Kippu—Compassion Is the New Currency," *GratisBasis* blog, July 4, 2013, http://gratisbasis.com/?p=498.

30. "Fureai Kippu."

31. Meghan O'Rourke, "The Shift Americans Must Make to Fight the Coronavirus," *Atlantic*, March 12, 2020, https://www.theatlantic.com/ideas/archive/2020/03/we-need-isolate-ourselves-during-coronavirus-outbreak/607840.

32. Claire Cain Miller, "Why Mothers' Choices About Work and Family Often Feel Like No Choice at All," *New York Times*, January 17, 2020, https://www.nytimes.com/2020/01/17/upshot/mothers-choices-work-family.html.

33. Megan Sholar, "Yes, Gillibrand and DeLauro Introduced a Family Leave Bill. More Important, Republicans Are Introducing Paid Leave Bills Too," *Washington Post*, February 20, 2019, https://www.washingtonpost.com/politics/2019/02/20/yes-gillibrand-delauro-introduced-family-leave-bill-more-important-republicans-are-introducing-paid-leave-bills-too.

34. Paid Leave for All (website), https://paidleaveforall.org/about-us.

35. Claire Cain Miller, Shane Goldmacher, and Thomas Kaplan, "Biden Announces $775 Billion Plan to Help Working Parents and Caregivers," *New York Times*, July 21, 2020, https://www.nytimes.com/2020/07/21/us/politics/biden-workplace-childcare.html.

36. Quoted in Chabeli Carranza, "America's First Female Recession," *The 19th*, August 2, 2020, https://19thnews.org/2020/08/americas-first-female-recession.

37. Kim Brooks, "Forget Pancakes. Pay Mothers," *New York Times*, May 8, 2020, https://www.nytimes.com/2020/05/08/opinion/sunday/women-housework-coronavirus-mothers-day.html.

38. "VA Caregiver Support," Department of Veterans Affairs website, https://www.caregiver.va.gov.

39. Tom Philpott, "Congress Opens VA Caregiver Plan to Thousands, Streamlines Access to Non-VA Care," *Tacoma News-Tribune*, May 24, 2018, https://www.thenewstribune.com/news/local/military/article211826254.html.

40. For a comprehensive overview of all the states' different Medicaid waiver programs, see www.medicaidwaiver.org.

41. See "Key Findings," Case for Inclusion 2020, prepared by staff from the ANCOR Foundation and United Cerebral Palsy (UCP), https://casefor inclusion.org/resources/key-findings.

42. Chris Gabbard, *A Life Beyond Reason: A Father's Memoir* (Boston: Beacon Press, 2019).

43. Chris Gabbard, interview with the author, June 2018.

44. Glenn, *Forced to Care*, 117. Chapter 4 of Glenn's book provides a detailed look at the legal history of obligating wives to care for their husbands without compensation.

45. Andrew Yang 2020 page, https://www.yang2020.com/what-is-freedom-dividend-faq.

46. Sarah Holder, "In Stockton, Early Clues Emerge About Impact of Guaranteed Income," *CityLab* (October 3, 2019), https://www.citylab.com/equity/2019/10/stockton-universal-basic-income-pilot-economic-empowerment/599152.

47. Melinda Gates, "How Rethinking Caregiving Could Play a Crucial Role in Restarting the Economy," *Washington Post*, May 7, 2020, https://www.washingtonpost.com/opinions/2020/05/07/melinda-gates-how-rethinking-caregiving-could-play-crucial-role-restarting-economy.

48. Libby Brittain, personal communication with the author, September 2020; https://www.quiltcanhelp.com.

49. Boyer, *The Undying*, 288.

50. Mia Birdsong, *How We Show Up: Reclaiming Family, Friendship,and Community* (New York: Hachette, 2020), 13.

51. Birdsong, *How We Show Up*, 22–23.

INDEX